Diverse Medicine

Building a Stronger and Healthier Nation

Dr. Dale Okorodudu, MD

White Coats Publishing

THIS BOOK IS DEDICATED TO:

My wife, Janai...thank you for always supporting me

My children...I hope daddy makes you proud

My patients...thank you for allowing me to care for you

God...thank you for everything

Book Contents

1. Speak Up   1

2. Achieving Excellence, Not Just Equity   17

3. Benefits of a More Diverse Workforce   39

4. Racism in Medicine   69

5. Empowering Communities   85

6. Rethinking Medical School Admissions   107

7. Diversifying Academic Medicine   123

8. Reducing Attrition   141

9. A Legacy of Unity   159

Chapter 1

SPEAK UP

"SPEAK UP FOR THOSE who cannot speak for themselves, for the rights of all who are destitute. Speak up and judge fairly; defend the rights of the poor and needy."
-Proverbs 31: 8-9

Standing outside the sliding glass door of my patient's room, a whirlwind of emotions swirled within me, weighing me down with a heavy sense of sadness. As a young clinician, I had this hopeful belief in our healthcare system, thinking it would provide fair chances and access to life-saving treatments, especially in the land of the free, the United States. But I soon learned what we hope for isn't always the case.

Mr. J, a patient on our cardiology service, was a remarkable man, fighting to survive against an enemy too well-known for many Americans. This enemy was congestive heart failure, and Mr. J was battling with all his might. Clenching on to every breath, he was determined to win the war and to leave the hospital with a second shot at life. His determination was contagious, and I became a fan. Like David facing Goliath, the little guy was in the thick of war, and I was rooting for the underdog.

As his medical team, we were also giving our all. Day in and day out, putting our minds together, ensuring we made the best decisions possible for Mr. J. This gave me great hope that he would walk out of the hospital. He had a dedicated team of healthcare providers looking out for his best interest. As the days passed, it became evident that Mr. J needed more than medications. Our intravenous therapies and cardiac-specific diets could only do so much. What Mr. J needed was a new heart. Having come this far, I knew we'd bring him through the finish line. He'd fought so hard, and we couldn't let him down now. Finally, the day came when we all realized our efforts seemed futile, and the last feasible option would be a heart transplant.

The next morning during patient rounds, I was invigorated with energy, believing he'd get his fair shot and, ultimately, a new heart. But that didn't happen. It hit me like a ton of bricks, and suddenly everything felt heavy, like the air thickened into a dense, suffocating cloud of despair. The moment had finally come for Mr. J to get a thorough evaluation for a heart transplant, but he was turned down because of social concerns. Time seemed to stop as I grappled with the weight of the decision and what it meant for our patient's life.

As I recall, the conversation about Mr. J being a heart transplant candidate was shockingly brief, leaving me with a lingering sense of missed opportunities and rushed judgments. This decision was made right there, at the patient's bedside, without further consultation or advancement to the transplant committee. I couldn't help but question if we, as his medical team, had given him a fair shot at life. Here he was, a man who had lived several decades on this planet, and we spent less than a few minutes discussing his candidacy for a transplant. Did we explore all possible options to ensure his well-being? Or did biases creep into our decision-making process, clouding our judgment without us even realizing it?

Being a Black man like Mr. J, I couldn't ignore the persistent thought that race may have played a part in all this. I desperately wanted to believe that wasn't true and race had nothing to do with it, but the doubts kept nagging at me. Would Mr. J have received a more thorough evaluation if his cardiologist shared the same racial background? Was there an unfair disparity in treatment outcomes because of biases deeply ingrained in our healthcare system? Should I have spoken up? Yes, I was a young clinician in training; however, a life was at stake. Or was I overthinking the entire situation? Could it simply be that they were right? My supervising doctors had years of experience beyond me, and perhaps that's all there was to it; he had social concerns that prohibited him from receiving a transplant. I don't know the answer, but these questions have haunted me, leaving me with greater responsibility and unease for our healthcare system. These instances have been the genesis for my efforts to leave the field of medicine better than I found it.

Such situations and questions inspired me to start my non-profit organization, DiverseMedicine Inc., in 2011. Our mission is straightforward, to increase diversity in the medical workforce and ensure every patient has a fair shot at life, regardless of race or social status. Over the years, I have worked alongside amazing individuals from all over the country who share our goals. We have mentored students, educated parents, influenced policymakers, and much more. The lessons learned along the journey have resulted in this book.

The Bible speaks to the importance of justice and fairness. Proverbs 31:8-9 says, "Speak up for those who cannot speak for themselves, for the rights of all who are destitute. Speak up and judge fairly; defend the rights of the poor and needy." These words have inspired me and become our organization's guiding principle. We believe every patient deserves to be heard and have a fair shot at life. Why? Because this is right.

Another key point in my journey came in 2021 when I had the incredible privilege of spearheading the production of a groundbreaking and landmark documentary called "Black Men in White Coats." This film represented the culmination of years of unwavering dedication and tireless efforts to increase Black men's representation in the medical field. Our collective goal was to create a powerful message that would echo across the nation, and the overwhelming praise, awards, and recognition we received following the film's release left me humbled and profoundly grateful.

One of the most remarkable achievements of the documentary was its widespread screening at most medical schools across the United States. This extraordinary opportunity allowed me to engage in profound conversations with medical school deans, presidents, and influential leaders within the field. I seized this platform to challenge them, urging them to proactively increase Black men's representation within their institutions. While the subsequent increase in Black men applying to medical school in the following years may have been modest, it was an encouraging step in the right direction. Many acknowledged the impact of our efforts and credited them as a significant contributing factor. However, we recognized that this progress remained insufficient to unlock the full potential of our healthcare system.

When I first embarked on the Black Men in White Coats movement in 2013, I faced skepticism and doubt from those who questioned the true significance of diversity in healthcare. Some argued that healthcare leadership merely sought to meet their diversity quotas without a genuine commitment to fostering inclusivity and reaping the positive outcomes it brings. Their words lingered in my mind for years, causing me to question the depth of our collective commitment to change. Yet, as I embarked on my journey, traversing the country to present our documentary in both virtual and physical settings, a profound truth became evident—I discovered that people truly do care. Hospital executives, deans, and the community at large; they cared! Their faces would light up during our discussions, and the questions they asked were challenging, with genuine intent for advancement. They cared! This realization filled me with a renewed sense of purpose, motivating me to complete this book that had been brewing in my mind for over a decade.

Throughout writing this book, I have continued to be humbled and uplifted by the steady stream of individuals seeking guidance on how they and their institutions can contribute to transforming our healthcare system through the power of diversity. These interactions serve as an affirmation that, despite those who may dismiss the importance of diversity in healthcare, there is a multitude of individuals who fervently believe in its intrinsic value. It has strengthened my confidence in America's medical system and its practitioners, who entered their respective fields fueled by a profound and unwavering passion for making a difference in people's lives. And most importantly, it has instilled a sense of faith in you, the reader, who has dedicated your time and attention to engage with the vital discussions presented in this book.

As our nation becomes increasingly diverse and the power of social media brings the flaws of our healthcare system into sharp focus, the need for diversity in healthcare has become more evident. The urgency for individual and institutional guidance resulting in action has never been more paramount. It is my hope that this book will serve as a compass, directing us toward a future where our healthcare system truly reflects the needs of the rich tapestry of our society, where every individual receives equitable and compassionate care, and where the transformative power of diversity flourishes to its fullest potential. Together, let us embark on this collective journey, driven by the unwavering belief that a more inclusive healthcare system is not just an aspiration but an essential requirement for the well-being and prosperity of all.

The War Against Diversity

Diversity has become a sensitive topic, often met with resistance and discomfort. The mere mention of it frequently triggers a reaction, one of protection, as if parents want to shield their children from its discussion. But why is diversity so polarizing? The answer lies in the ongoing war against diversity efforts, with supporters fighting not just for opportunities to improve our systems but also against the ideals of some who oppose it. In simple terms, diversity is under attack.

Before delving deeper, it is crucial to establish a common ground. We should all strive for the same outcome – building and maintaining an infrastructure that ensures the best possible care for everyone. Even if we have different approaches and preferences for achieving it, we should be united in this goal. Sadly, instead of working as a dream team, it sometimes feels like we are caught up in a royal rumble, a rivalry that spans generations, hindering our progress toward a shared vision.

America's history is intricately woven with the issue of race. From the dark times of slavery to the era of Jim Crow laws, race relations have always been complex and deeply rooted in our society. In recent years, diversity has ignited intense debates, with some perceiving it as an assault on a nation's history and meritocracy. In contrast, others view it as a necessary catalyst for societal advancement.

This war against diversity presents itself in various forms, including legal challenges to implementing diversity initiatives and the dismantling of current efforts at the federal level. A prominent example is the Fisher v. University of Texas at Austin case, where Abigail Fisher argued that her white race led to her denial of admission to the university. Although she ultimately lost the case, it set a modern precedent for challenging affirmative action and other diversity programs.

During the Trump administration, the battle against diversity escalated. The Department of Justice investigated alleged discrimination against non-underrepresented minority applicants in colleges and universities. Additionally, the administration revoked Obama-era guidance on diversity initiatives in schools. Simultaneously, a new narrative emerged in the media, with pundits and politicians claiming that diversity programs were discriminatory and unfair.

Consequently, these actions had a chilling effect on diversity programs and initiatives nationwide. Companies and organizations became apprehensive about implementing diversity programs, fearing legal repercussions or negative media attention. In many instances, diversity hires and promotions declined, stalling or even reversing progress toward a more equitable society.

Just yesterday, while walking out of my local gym, I saw a commercial on TV. It went something like this. "Diversity Equity and Inclusion policies are discriminating against people and causing them to be turned down from the jobs they deserve. If you have been unlawfully denied employment based on your race, contact our law offices now." The commercial's provocative statements shed light on a growing concern. It implied that the policies designed to foster diversity and inclusion in the workforce could sometimes inadvertently lead to unfair and discriminatory outcomes. In other words, they would perpetuate the flaws they were created to eradicate.

In pursuing a more equitable society, where do we draw the line between creating equal opportunities and ensuring fair treatment for all? Can DEI (Diversity, Equity, & Inclusion) policies inadvertently contribute to unintended consequences, such as reverse discrimination or the exclusion of qualified individuals? The advertisement unintentionally highlighted a delicate balance that needs to be struck. How do we acknowledge the importance of diversity and rectify the results of discriminatory atrocities of the past while, at the same time, not penalizing those currently working hard to earn their way based on merit?

To fully understand the complexities at play, it is essential to recognize the origins and purpose of DEI policies. They emerged as a response to historical inequalities, seeking to fix systemic biases that have long plagued our society. The aim was to level the playing field, ensuring that individuals from diverse backgrounds had equal access to employment opportunities, career advancement, and workplace inclusivity.

However, as with any transformative endeavor, implementing DEI policies has faced its fair share of challenges. Critics argue that some organizations might inadvertently prioritize race or ethnicity over merit and qualifications in their quest for diversity. Concerns have been raised that qualified individuals, regardless of their racial background, may be denied opportunities solely based on an attempt to meet diversity quotas. Rather than delivering meaningful solutions, DEI policies may, in fact, be weakening the workforce for the sake of inclusivity.

As the commercial underscored, individuals who feel unjustly excluded from employment due to their race or ethnicity may perceive DEI policies as a barrier rather than a solution. Some consider DEI initiatives as legitimate attacks on merit and, in turn, our nation. On the radical end, a few would even consider these efforts intentionally anti-American. However, the reality is that diversity does not threaten meritocracy but rather enhances it. Uniformity within a workforce can hinder our ability to identify unique qualities, character traits, and skill sets that are merit derived and add value to society. If all I've ever heard is a string quartet, how would I appreciate the value of a master pianist? How could I determine the commitment necessary to reach that level, and how that commitment could translate into a better, more harmonic ensemble? Diversity in and of itself enhances our ability to identify and judge merit. Regarding healthcare specifically, we can cultivate a pool of healthcare providers and researchers who bring unique perspectives and ideas by promoting diversity. This, in turn, leads to better healthcare outcomes for individuals of all races and ethnicities.

Ultimately, the war on diversity in the medical field is not a clash between different races or ideologies but a battle for the future of healthcare in America. This itself is intertwined with the future of the nation as a whole. And to secure this future, we must collaborate to promote diversity and inclusivity across all aspects of healthcare, ranging from hiring practices to research initiatives. Contrary to some beliefs, it's worth noting that this can be achieved in a relatively fair manner. The real challenge lies in determining what constitutes fairness and developing criteria for what constitutes true merit. Once we can address these questions and incorporate them into our decision-making processes, we will be on the right track to improving not just healthcare but all American industries.

America's Health Paradox

The United States is widely regarded as one of the most advanced countries in the world, with a thriving economy, cutting-edge technology, and a high standard of living. However, when it comes to health, our country seems to be falling behind. Despite spending more on healthcare than the vast majority of countries in the world, Americans as a whole are not getting healthier. In fact, according to recent statistics, the health of the average American is getting worse, with increasing rates of chronic medical conditions such as obesity, diabetes, and heart disease.

According to a report by the World Health Organization, the United States ranks 37th in the world in terms of healthcare outcomes, despite spending more on healthcare than any other country. Consider these key healthcare statistics at the time of this writing:

- The United States spends over $3.6 trillion on healthcare annually, more than any other country globally.

- Life expectancy in the United States is lower than in many other developed countries, at 76.1 years.

- The United States has the highest rate of obesity in the world, with 36.2% of the population classified as obese.

- The United States also has high rates of chronic diseases such as diabetes and heart disease, often linked to poor diet and lifestyle choices.

Paramount to America's floundering medical system are healthcare disparities. These disparities refer to differences in health outcomes and healthcare access based on race, ethnicity, socioeconomic status, and geography. For example, African Americans and Hispanics are more likely to suffer from chronic diseases like diabetes and heart disease than whites. They are also more likely to lack access to quality healthcare. In addition, rural areas often have fewer healthcare resources than urban areas, leading to disparities in access to care for those residing in such locales. As long as these disparities exist and continue to progress, our nation's health will remain on life support.

A Prescription for Diversity

I must state this clearly: your skin color does not determine how great of a clinician you can become. If all the doctors in the world were of one race, I wouldn't have a problem with that as long as they could practice with complete compassion, fairness, non-bias, and love towards everyone. However, achieving that level of practice is extremely challenging, and I don't believe society is currently capable of it. In fact, I don't believe human nature allows us to fully achieve it. As long as self-interest exists, disparities will persist. This is precisely why we need adequate diversity in the healthcare workforce.

This is what I believe; diversity in the medical workforce is the key to creating the most effective healthcare system we can design. Studies have shown that patients are more likely to receive better care when treated by healthcare providers who share their racial or ethnic backgrounds. We'll cover this in more detail shortly. In addition, a diverse healthcare workforce is better equipped to understand and address the medical needs of different communities, including those historically facing healthcare disparities.

Knowing this, it's bothersome that the US medical workforce remains largely homogeneous, with a notable lack of diversity among doctors, nurses, and allied healthcare professionals. According to the Association of American Medical Colleges, only 5% of practicing physicians in the United States are African American, and only 7% are Hispanic. Further complicating matters, women and minorities are underrepresented in healthcare leadership roles. It's past due time the American healthcare system is treated with a dose of diversity. The ideas put forth in this book are ones I believe have the potential to transform and elevate our healthcare system to unprecedented heights.

I hope every healthcare executive, dean, educator, and decision-maker will consider this book required reading as we work together to improve American health. Let's build a stronger and healthier nation!

Author Notes: Watch our Black Men In White Coats Documentary at www.BMWCmovie.com

Chapter 2

ACHIEVING EXCELLENCE, NOT JUST EQUITY

"THE SANDLOT," A CLASSIC film from the days of my childhood, holds a special place in my heart. It tells the story of Smalls, a timid child looking to make friends in a new neighborhood. One day while on the diamond, the boys desperately need a baseball to play with. Smalls, who doesn't know much about the sport, innocently lends his father's prized baseball to the group of neighborhood boys for a sandlot game. Unbeknownst to him, the legendary Babe Ruth had autographed the ball, making it an invaluable treasure.

As fate would have it, Smalls hits his first home run during the game, but the ball lands deep within the neighboring yard, guarded by a fearsome dog known as "The Beast." Determined to retrieve the precious ball, the group of friends embarks on a series of thrilling adventures and comical misadventures. Along the way, they encounter numerous obstacles, face their fears, and learn important life lessons.

In one pivotal moment, after a particularly disastrous attempt to recover the ball, the character Victor DiMattia, with a hint of remorse in his voice, utters the profound words, "We've been going about this all wrong... I blame myself." This heartfelt admission reflects the genuine bonds of friendship forged among the boys and their shared responsibility for their actions.

This scene in "The Sandlot" encapsulates a universal truth that resonates beyond the film's nostalgic storyline. It reminds us that sometimes, in pursuing our goals or resolving a challenge, no matter how much effort we've already put in, we must take a step back and evaluate our approach honestly. In doing this, we may realize that our approach has been suboptimal. In such cases, we must take ownership of shortcomings, learn from them, and adapt our strategies accordingly.

I must clarify one thing before moving forward. The work of many who have come before me in diversifying the medical workforce needs to be acknowledged. By no means would I suggest they were misguided or consider their efforts suboptimal. As a matter of fact, I fear what the medical landscape would have looked like had they not been so committed to the purpose. It's likely the status of diversity within the workforce would be much worse than it is today. The thought of that is quite frightening to me. With that in mind, I'm grateful for those who came before me and those working alongside me. The Bible tells us that it is right to give honor to whom honor is due, so I tip my hat and thank these trailblazers who have carried us this far.

Now back to the Sandlot. Just as DiMattia and his baseball crew had to reevaluate their strategies to retrieve the coveted baseball, we must confront the stark reality that persistent health disparities are exacerbated by our failure to cultivate a truly diverse and inclusive medical workforce. Using statistics around Black men attending medical school as an example, the dismal numbers were grossly stagnant for 40-plus years. How in the world is that possible? It's difficult to fathom that the amount of resources we poured into increasing racial and ethnic diversity in healthcare over those 40 years resulted in grossly no increase in the number of Black men entering the field. As hard as it is for me to say this, we're failing in this mission.

When I use the word "our" before failure, I'm referring to all of us working in the medical field. This is a shared responsibility. When my household is messy, I call upon everyone to help clean it up. This includes my three children, my wife, and myself. Like the famous song from "High School Musical," we're all in this together. Everyone inhabiting the space has a part in cleaning things up. This realization compels us to reflect and ask ourselves that critical question: Have we been going about this all wrong? This is a challenging question as it's difficult to admit our shortcomings; however, it's worth consideration.

If I had to identify the single most important factor contributing to our lack of progression as it pertains to diversity in the medical field, I'd argue it's the lack of buy-in from key stakeholders and influencers. When I think about rectifying this issue, I'm reminded of one individual in particular.

Among my favorite books is Up From Slavery by Booker T. Washington. Washington, who would become a foremost leader in Black America and beyond, was born into slavery and, along with his family, gained freedom from the Emancipation Proclamation when he was nine. Eventually, he would attend Hampton Institute and work his way through school. At the young age of 25, he became the president of the Tuskegee Institute, now known as Tuskegee University.

Washington believed that Blacks should "cast down their buckets," as he put it in his famous Atlanta Compromise Speech. Basically, this meant working as hard as you can with what you have, and this work will elevate you in society. Simultaneously, unify with those in a position to uplift your community and demonstrate that when you do better, they do better as well. A rising tide lifts all boats. This, I believe, is where our modern-day efforts have fallen short. Those who pull the strings in health-care must also see how their boats will be lifted.

Nobody really states the obvious, but I'm going to do that right now. People with power want to keep their power. If I control the resources, why would I ever want to give that up if I'm in a position of power? Why would I give you the resources and opportunity to compete with me? Let's say we're playing a game, and I know all the rules win. Everything is set in my favor. Then you come along and try to change the rules to benefit you. Do you really think I will sit there and simply let you change the rules? No way. That is not happening. There are only two reasons I'd be amenable to a rule change. First, you must demonstrate that your rule change would also benefit me. Second, I'd have to come from a place of true love in my heart, valuing your needs as much as mine. We must achieve both of these to increase diversity in the medical field. We must demonstrate that diversity in healthcare is that tide that will lift all boats.

I'm convinced we can do just that. In general, a larger segment of the medical field and society would support diversity efforts if they better understood the mission and methods to achieve it. A significant factor contributing to its opposition is how the message is delivered. Many people wrongly assume that the main reason diversity is promoted in healthcare is only to address issues related to equity. Further complicating that, a poor understanding of healthcare equity could lead one to believe their resources are in jeopardy of being unfairly reallocated to other individuals. While equity is important, I believe it cannot be the primary message in championing diversity. Rather, the messaging should focus on its necessity to achieve excellence in healthcare. We shouldn't be saying diversity leads to excellence. Instead, the message should be we cannot achieve excellence without diversity. That nuance makes a monumental difference.

Defining Equity

Equity is a word commonly used without proper consideration of its true definition. Its concept refers to fairness, impartiality, and justice. In medical terms, the word is meant to ensure all patients receive appropriate access to healthcare services and resources regardless of their background, race, ethnicity, gender, or socioeconomic status. This also means that healthcare providers should strive to eliminate disparities or barriers preventing patients from accessing healthcare services.

It is important to note that while equity and equality are often used interchangeably, they are two distinct concepts. Equality refers to treating everyone equally, regardless of their needs or circumstances. In contrast, equity means treating everyone based on their needs and circumstances. Let's use an illustration to understand the difference between equity and equality in healthcare.

Consider Ashley, Bob, and Charlie, three patients with diabetes who all need to purchase medications to manage their blood glucose levels. Ashley is a vibrant Black woman who grew up in poverty. She was the child of a single teenage mother, and they struggled throughout her developmental years. Fortunately for Ashley, she had a loving mom who went to the extreme to ensure her daughter would be successful. Taking her to the library each Sunday, Ashley's mother helped her see the world beyond the streets of their housing projects.

Today, Ashley is a wealthy CEO and founder of a Fortune 500 company. When it comes time to pick up her medications from the pharmacy, Ashley can afford to buy them out of pocket without insurance. Her hemoglobin A1c, a measurement of diabetes control, is excellent at a normal level of 5.9.

Robert, a humble Hispanic man, is an attorney for a leading law firm. He has a good health insurance plan that covers the cost of his medication, but his diet isn't the best because he's always working to make ends meet. Bob is doing okay health-wise, with a hemoglobin A1c level of 7.4. Although insurance covers the cost of medications, his lifestyle isn't ideal for diabetes control.

On the other hand, Charlie, a humorous White man, was raised in one of America's wealthiest counties. His dad was a well-known doctor and provided for the family. Healthcare wasn't Charlie's thing, and he chose to pursue a career in technology, working for a videogame company as a software engineer. Unfortunately, Bob recently lost his insurance when he was laid off from his job due to a floundering economy. Now, he's struggling financially and can't afford the cost of his diabetes medications.

Furthermore, his lifestyle habits and diet are a mess. Charlie is simply focused on getting by on a day-to-day basis. When his doctor asks why his hemoglobin A1c is horrendous at 13.1, Charlie replies, "I'm just trying to survive and keep a roof over my family's head."

If we were to approach Ashley, Bob, and Charlie equally, they'd get the same financial support, medications, and resources to improve their lifestyle. The question is, would that be adequate? Or would that be fair? Whose level of need would you base the rationing on? On the other hand, treating our three patients in an equitable manner would allow us to consider each individual's specific needs. Ashley needs the least amount of support, and Charlie requires the most.

The Unfairness of Equity

"The hardest lesson in life is that life is unfair." – John F. Kennedy

Equity is often misconceived as synonymous with fairness, but their principles can diverge. While fairness emphasizes impartiality and honesty, equity operates on a different premise, reflecting a higher level of social consciousness. It recognizes that equal treatment may not always lead to the best outcomes for everyone involved.

Equity serves as a corrective factor to bridge gaps, not a foundational one. Its role is to offset the disadvantages plaguing individuals or groups due to various social, economic, or historical factors. In an ideal world, fairness would prevent these disadvantages from ever developing, ensuring everyone starts on an equal footing. However, in our imperfect reality, these disadvantages persist, significantly impacting people's lives and opportunities. That's where equity comes in, bridging the gap and providing necessary support to meet each individual's needs.

To illustrate the importance of equity, let's consider the role of parenting. As a father to three amazing yet unique children, I understand the importance of tailoring my approach to each of them. Discipline is necessary for all kids, but I don't discipline my children equally. Instead, I consider their personalities, ages, interests, and needs for further development. For instance, Tony may require a month's grounding, Jace may only need a firm one-minute scolding, while writing sentences may be sufficient for Debby. By recognizing and acknowledging their distinct needs, I treat my children equitably, not equally, to maximize their individual opportunities for success and happiness. The same is necessary for society at large. Simply put, some groups need more help than others. Some groups have been unfairly disadvantaged, and now the right thing to do is correct that via equity.

Getting equity right can be a real challenge. What's equitable for one person or group might not seem fair for another. Imagine you're the manager of a basketball team. Your team already has five players in the center position, but you need a point guard. Now, the league commissioner decides that every team should get an extra player on their team, but the player must be in the center position. This isn't good for you because you already have five centers. What you need is a point guard. While teams that lack centers might be happy with the new rule, it disadvantages your team. In this case, what you really want is equity. You want the commissioner to understand your team's specific needs and give you the right player to help you succeed. This example shows why it's important to consider individual circumstances and find equitable solutions tailored to each situation.

Keeping on the topic of basketball, let's look at how equity can serve as a corrective factor for the betterment of a system. The NBA draft lottery presents an intriguing system that employs the principle of equity to achieve long-term fairness. Historically, teams based in larger markets have garnered more attention and often enjoy greater success, both in terms of victories on the court and financial gains. However, the NBA recognizes that for the league to thrive in the long run, it cannot be dominated solely by these select teams. It is crucial to allow other teams to compete and have the opportunity to succeed.

To prevent a handful of teams from dominating year after year, the NBA implements a lottery raffle to determine the order in which teams are granted their draft picks. This is where we see equity at work. Teams that performed poorly in the previous season are allocated more raffle tickets, or in this case, raffle balls, for the lottery drawing. As a result, they possess higher mathematical odds of securing an earlier draft pick, increasing their chances of selecting a talented player who can potentially become a star and increase fanfare in their market. This leads to more revenue for the NBA as a whole. Equity is a corrective factor, optimizing the overall NBA system to benefit all teams, not just a privileged few. This concept extends beyond the NBA and applies to various systems in life. Equity creates vital opportunities, not only for individuals but for society as a whole.

Amidst this understanding of equity, it is crucial to recognize the often-overlooked aspect of love and charity required to achieve it. Equity goes beyond mere equality because it is rooted in genuine care and concern. It involves meeting individuals where they are, addressing their needs, and approaching them compassionately. This perspective emphasizes that everyone deserves to be treated with dignity, regardless of their starting point. By embracing equity, we cultivate a culture of generosity and empathy where individuals willingly contribute their time, resources, and talents to support those who are less fortunate.

Relevant to the spirit of equity, 2 Corinthians 9:7 reminds us of the voluntary nature of giving. The verse states, "Each one must give as he has decided in his heart, not reluctantly or under compulsion, for God loves a cheerful giver." It highlights the importance of genuine generosity and the challenge of promoting equity without imposing its responsibility on others. This verse underscores the significance of nurturing a culture of voluntary giving, where individuals willingly contribute to the betterment of society and the well-being of others.

In healthcare, equity serves as a powerful tool for rectifying historical injustices and fostering positive health outcomes for all individuals. It recognizes the systemic barriers and discrimination that underrepresented communities have faced and seeks to address these disparities by allocating additional resources and support where needed. Achieving equity in healthcare necessitates a collective effort involving healthcare providers, policymakers, community leaders, and patients. Collaboration among these stakeholders is crucial to dismantle existing inequities and promote a more just healthcare system. It requires active listening to diverse perspectives, acknowledging the lived experiences of marginalized communities, and engaging in meaningful dialogue.

By understanding the unique challenges and barriers different populations face, we can develop comprehensive solutions that address systemic issues such as limited access to care, discriminatory practices, and bias within healthcare delivery. Moreover, achieving equity in healthcare extends beyond simply addressing immediate concerns. It involves implementing sustainable strategies that promote long-term improvements in health outcomes for all individuals. This may include initiatives to expand access to healthcare services, enhance health education and awareness in underserved communities, and advocate for policies prioritizing equitable resource and opportunity distribution.

By working together to promote equity in healthcare, we can create a system that ensures everyone has an opportunity to lead a healthy and fulfilling life. This requires an ongoing commitment to identify and rectify disparities, foster inclusivity, and empower individuals to actively participate in their healthcare journey. Ultimately, the pursuit of equity in healthcare is not only a moral imperative but also a fundamental step towards building a healthier society for all. Someone once said, "Life is unfair, but it's our response to that unfairness that defines us." Utilizing equity is our opportunity to respond to that unfairness.

Aiming For Excellence

I've always been troubled by the notion that equity and excellence cannot coexist. Although not openly admitted, it is apparent that this viewpoint is pervasive in our society. We witness this perspective manifesting in lawsuits against affirmative action, where the argument suggests that the most qualified candidates are being disregarded in favor of promoting diversity.

This argument falsely assumes that excellence is being compromised in pursuing diversity. However, this reasoning is flawed as it fails to recognize that diversity strives to elevate genuine excellence.

The misconception lies in an incomplete understanding of the relationship between diversity and excellence. Embracing diversity does not diminish or undermine excellence but enhances it. When individuals from diverse backgrounds, experiences, and perspectives come together, it fosters a rich tapestry of ideas, innovation, and creativity. By valuing diversity, we create an environment that nurtures excellence in its truest sense.

Excellence is a maintained state of high standards which exceed expectations. It is something that everybody wants. Not everybody cares about equity and disparities, but everyone loves excellence. With this in mind, I am of the opinion that when working to enhance diversity in the medical field, the outcome of focus should not stop at equity and eradicating health disparities. Instead, the focus should be elevating our healthcare system to a place of excellence.

While many people think diversity is only a problem for minority communities, the truth is that it affects all Americans, regardless of their race, ethnicity, or culture. The very nature of the word is meant to be inclusive of everyone. Should we fail to appreciate this truth, we risk irrevocable consequences. This goes beyond healthcare, as we've seen the importance of diversity in other fields.

Let's start with the tech industry, which has long been criticized for its lack of diversity. While this issue was initially seen as a problem for women and people of color, it eventually became clear that it was also a problem for the industry as a whole. The lack of diversity in tech has had far-reaching consequences. With a narrow focus on certain types of products and services, the sector failed to cater to the needs of a diverse user base. This limited perspective resulted in missed opportunities for innovation and growth. By excluding diverse voices and perspectives, the industry hindered its progress and alienated potential users who felt marginalized and underserved. This lack of inclusivity had a detrimental impact on the industry's reputation and, in some instances, eroded public trust.

Next, let's talk about money. The finance industry has encountered its fair share of challenges potentially stemming from a lack of diversity. This has resulted in a limited focus on specific market segments and diminished economic opportunities for certain groups. Within this space are multiple glaring examples of the potential consequences when a company fails to cultivate diversity. One investment bank specifically stands out to me. For anonymity, I'll call them "Bank ABC ." As a major investment bank, Bank ABC experienced a dramatic downfall during the 2008 financial crisis, largely attributable to its heavy investments in risky mortgage-backed securities.

An issue with Bank ABC lay in its absence of diversity within the workforce, which may have hampered its ability to accurately assess and navigate the risks associated with complex financial products. With a sub-optimally diverse employee base, the company faced difficulties appreciating the potential hazards and vulnerabilities in the housing market.

The organization's absence of varied voices and perspectives perpetuated a culture of conformity, inhibiting critical examination of prevailing assumptions. This narrow mindset likely hindered the identification of systemic risks and the implementation of effective risk management strategies.

Bank ABC encountered severe losses as the housing market deteriorated and the subprime mortgage crisis unfolded. The firm was heavily exposed to toxic assets and faced substantial challenges in meeting its financial obligations. Ultimately, Bank ABC had to be acquired by another institution with assistance from the Federal Reserve, signifying its position as one of the significant casualties of the financial crisis.

The entertainment industry has also been heavily criticized for its lack of diversity and accurate representation of diverse voices and experiences. This has sparked important discussions about the need for greater inclusion within the industry. When diversity is not adequately embraced, the entertainment industry unintentionally perpetuates stereotypes and misses out on the chance to tell authentic and meaningful stories from various perspectives.

The absence of diversity in the entertainment industry leads to a limited range of narratives and characters portrayed on screen, reinforcing narrow and often distorted depictions of various communities. This perpetuation of stereotypes harms marginalized groups and hinders the exploration of untold stories and unique viewpoints that could resonate with diverse audiences.

By fostering greater diversity, the entertainment industry can break free from the confines of traditional norms and tap into a vast array of narratives that truly reflect the diversity of our society. This inclusivity enriches storytelling and creates opportunities for talented individuals from marginalized communities to contribute their creative vision and expertise.

Acknowledging the significance of representation, there is a growing demand for diverse voices and stories in film, television, and other forms of entertainment. Audiences increasingly seek genuine and inclusive content that mirrors their lived experiences and diverse perspectives. Embracing diversity drives social progress and presents a considerable commercial opportunity for the entertainment industry, as it can attract broader audiences and foster deeper audience engagement.

Now, let's bring it back to healthcare. We'll discuss this throughout the entirety of the book, but briefly, let's touch on a recent example where diversity brought us to excellence. The COVID pandemic was among the most frightening crises we've seen since the AIDS epidemic. As a world, we were faced with a seemingly unstoppable enemy, invisible to the naked eye. This coronavirus variant was having its way with us, and it seemed there was nothing we could do about it.

Among the major concerns in the United States was the virus appeared to devastate minority communities at a disproportionate rate. It should be noted that there are several medical conditions that impact minorities with a higher incidence. However, it's the ones that can easily spread out of the minority communities which seem to garner the most attention and immediate action. COVID is one of those. As the spread approached critical speed, it became obvious we needed mechanisms to slow the pace, especially in minority communities. This, in turn, would hopefully decrease infection rates for everyone else.

During this process, excellence via diversity was witnessed as minority doctors and healthcare professionals across the country were called upon. These individuals were heavily relied on to enter these communities, not only to provide healthcare but also to gain the trust of their constituents and communicate credible health guidance around concepts such as vaccination and "social distancing." The result of this was one of America's most excellent moments in healthcare as we watched healthcare providers from diverse backgrounds all come together to take on the monster that was and is COVID. Diversity was necessary for us to achieve this level of excellence. Without it, who knows the extent of devastation COVID would have left us with.

As we navigated the COVID-19 storm, the impact of diversity and excellence in healthcare became ever more apparent. Beyond the medical frontlines, we witnessed individuals from various backgrounds collaborating to combat this ruthless virus. It wasn't just about healthcare providers; it was also about community leaders, activists, and everyday heroes who stepped up to protect the vulnerable. By embracing diversity, we found strength in unity, fostering a sense of understanding and empathy among us all. The pandemic taught us that when we stand together, acknowledging the unique challenges faced by different communities, we become more resilient and effective in facing adversity. This revelation serves as a profound reminder that embracing diversity in healthcare is not just essential for emergencies; it's a vital ingredient for a healthier and stronger nation, no matter the circumstances we encounter.

That's the critical message of this book. Diversity is not just about equality and equity; it is about excellence. Once society can come to terms with this, progress in healthcare and a multitude of industries can be made to extents yet seen. By embracing diversity, healthcare providers can tap into a wealth of knowledge, experiences, and perspectives, enhancing clinical outcomes and patient satisfaction. Ultimately, this is not a challenge that solely affects marginalized groups but rather a collective responsibility that demands collaboration and concerted efforts from all healthcare institutions. By working together, we can build a healthcare system that embodies excellence, equality, and inclusivity for the benefit of everyone.

Chapter 3

Benefits of a More Diverse Workforce

THE UNITED STATES HEALTHCARE system is one of the most advanced in the world, with cutting-edge technology, innovative treatments, and highly skilled healthcare providers. Yet, despite these advancements, we still face significant challenges, including a lack of diversity in the medical field. According to a 2023 Association of American Medical Colleges report, just 5.7% of physicians in the United States are Black, and only 6.9% are Hispanic. This lack of diversity also extends to other healthcare professions, with Black and Hispanic nurses, pharmacists, and other healthcare professionals also underrepresented.

The US medical system has been subject to criticism for many years. This goes beyond the professional realm and even into pop culture. Sean Carter, a well-known American rapper, and businessman who goes by the stage name Jay Z, once said, "The health care system and the health care plan in America is a joke. It's really a joke; it's not designed to help us. It's not designed for us to get healthy. It's designed for us to get sick... they don't care about poor people." Regardless of whether his statement is accurate, the perception that healthcare is not designed to benefit everyone but rather to benefit certain groups highlights a major issue in our medical system.

For nearly two decades, since my days as an undergraduate student, my argument has been the same; a more ethnically diverse medical workforce can improve the healthcare system. A major misconception around this topic is that diversity among healthcare providers only benefits minorities and the poor. However, in reality, diversity in healthcare can benefit all Americans. From a health perspective, having a more diverse workforce allows a better understanding of cultural beliefs, practice norms, and values that may impact a patient's health. This leads to more effective communication and better health outcomes for all patients, not just minorities and the poor. We'll dive into health outcomes shortly, but let's start with what talks, money.

Economic Impact of Diversity In Healthcare

"Money doesn't discriminate, neither should we." – Unknown

Here's one thing I know; if you want to get people listening, talk about money. It's one thing that we can all relate to, and we should be on the same page as it pertains to strengthening our nation's economy.

Here's a fun fact. Well, maybe not so fun, but it's important. In 2021, the Center for Medicare and Medicaid Services reported that healthcare expenditures account for approximately 18% of the United States' gross domestic product. In dollars, this equates to nearly $4 trillion. That's a lot of money! To put this number in perspective, spending $1 million daily would take you almost 10,959 years to spend $4 trillion.

Money plays a significant role in every industry, including healthcare. Despite the idealized image of medicine as an altruistic and selfless field, financial considerations hold considerable influence. Recognizing the economic advantages of fostering greater diversity within the healthcare workforce becomes crucial in this context. In 2017, the National Bureau of Economic Research conducted an extensive study that revealed a strong link between workforce diversity, improved healthcare outcomes, and reduced costs. This study analyzed a vast dataset spanning from 1992 to 2010, encompassing over 1.8 million hospital admissions in Florida. The findings were eye-opening, showing that hospitals with a more diverse medical staff, comprising doctors, nurses, and other healthcare professionals, witnessed significant reductions in healthcare spending. In fact, the study estimated that a more diverse workforce could potentially lead to a 20% reduction in healthcare costs.

The financial advantages of diversity in healthcare stem from several key factors. One factor is providing high-quality care that acknowledges patients' unique needs and cultural backgrounds. A diverse medical team, with individuals bringing various perspectives, experiences, and cultural competencies, can deliver more personalized and effective care. This tailored approach helps avoid unnecessary or ineffective procedures, resulting in substantial cost savings.

Moreover, diverse healthcare teams are better equipped to address health disparities and provide culturally sensitive care. Effective communication with patients from different backgrounds, understanding their healthcare challenges, and delivering appropriate interventions can reduce healthcare costs associated with preventable complications or prolonged treatments.

Additionally, diversity within medical teams fosters innovation and creativity in healthcare delivery. With a mix of perspectives and problem-solving approaches, diverse teams are more likely to develop new treatment strategies, techniques, and technologies. This spirit of innovation improves efficiency, streamlines processes, and can ultimately contribute to cost savings within the healthcare system.

A concrete example illustrating the cost-reducing potential of diversity can be observed in a study conducted by the University of Michigan in 2003. The university established a diversity council intending to promote diversity in healthcare. The council focused on recruiting healthcare providers from underrepresented communities and enhancing cultural competency training for all healthcare staff. As a direct result of these efforts, the hospital achieved a remarkable 15% reduction in nursing turnover, resulting in approximately $1 million in annual savings.

Ultimately, cost savings in healthcare can be attained through increased system efficiency, influenced by various factors such as early disease detection and treatment, patient compliance, decreased staff turnover, and innovation in diagnostic and therapeutic technologies. With each component, increased diversity catalyzes improvement, fostering a financially sustainable healthcare system that delivers better outcomes for all individuals.

Racial Concordance and Trust

Recently, I watched the movie "Devotion" starring Jonathan Majors. In the film, Majors portrays the black naval aviator Jesse Brown, who battles racial discrimination while striving to become the best pilot he can be. In a poignant scene, Majors's character confides in his wingman, Hudner, played by actor Glen Powell. He confesses his insecurities about learning to fly a new plane and being afraid to land it. Hudner then advises him to trust the white Landing Safety Officer (LSO), who uses bright flags to guide pilots to a safe landing. In response, Majors's character answers, "Hard to believe that the LSO won't crash my black [explicit] on purpose." Hearing those words, I immediately appreciated how that sentiment reflects a disturbing reality many underrepresented minorities face when seeking healthcare.

Mr. Johnson, a former patient, is the perfect example of this. His mistrust and fear of the healthcare system were deeply rooted in his personal experiences and the historical context of medical mistreatment towards marginalized communities. As a physician, I understood the importance of addressing his concerns and building trust in his healthcare team. Leaning close, I made eye contact, empathizing with his apprehension. "I can see you're worried, Mr. Johnson. It's completely understandable, given the history of mistreatment that some communities have faced. However, I want you to know that we are committed to providing you with the best care possible. Our priority is your well-being, and we value your trust."

Mr. Johnson's tense posture relaxed slightly as he cautiously listened to my words. His fear slowly gave way to a glimmer of hope as he recognized my genuine concern for his welfare. As our conversation progressed, I listened attentively to Mr. Johnson's fears and frustrations, validating his experiences and emotions. Through open and honest communication, I aimed to bridge the gap of mistrust and establish a foundation of understanding and collaboration. Over time, with continued reassurance, Mr. Johnson developed a sense of trust in his healthcare team, a sense of trust in us. He became more open to adhering to his prescribed medications and following our recommended treatment plans. The transformation was beautiful.

This example highlights the significance of trust-building efforts in healthcare, particularly when patients harbor deep-seated mistrust due to historical and personal experiences. By acknowledging and addressing these concerns, we as healthcare providers can work towards fostering a supportive and inclusive environment where every patient feels safe, heard, and valued.

Although I've modified certain story details for patient anonymity, it is disheartening to acknowledge that conversations like these are not uncommon. Many individuals from marginalized communities carry deep-rooted mistrust toward the medical system, stemming from historical atrocities passed down through generations. They have witnessed their parents and ancestors struggle to receive adequate care within a system they perceive as not advocating for them. This, in turn, leads to troubled interactions with the healthcare system.

While I am aware of the negative implications of stereotypes, I also recognize that they can be ethically employed in certain contexts to benefit patients. Racial concordance in healthcare is one such example. This concept refers to aligning a patient's race with their healthcare provider's. Ideally, race should not play a role in patient care, and we should strive to move beyond its significance. However, given the current state of our society and the existing disparities, research is finding that racial concordance plays a crucial role in healthcare outcomes and patient experiences.

The United States is a diverse melting pot of cultures, ethnicities, and races. As our nation continues to evolve and become more diverse, our healthcare system should reflect this diversity. The growing diversity within our population corresponds to an equally diverse array of medical conditions that must be addressed by a medical workforce capable of accommodating these changes. We must embrace inclusivity, recognize each patient's unique needs, and strive to provide equitable care to all individuals, regardless of their racial or ethnic background. Furthermore, it's important to recognize that certain groups require more attention to elevate their health to par.

Multiple studies have demonstrated that patients' trust in their physicians significantly impacts their health outcomes. Patients like Mr. Johnson may place greater trust in a physician who shares their racial background based on the color of their skin. This unsettling reality has been corroborated by reputable research, including a study published by the National Bureau of Economic Research in 2018. The study revealed that Black men were more likely to adhere to preventive health screenings and receive flu shots when their doctors were also Black. Analyzing data from a large healthcare organization, the research found that race concordance led to a 29% increase in the probability of Black men accessing preventive services. Furthermore, the study discovered that Black male patients held a more favorable perception of their doctors and felt a genuine sense of care when their physicians were racially concordant.

The notion that we can enhance patients' health by providing doctors who share their racial background is a compelling impetus to advocate for greater diversity in the medical workforce. Mistrust is a tangible and consequential issue, capable of making the difference between life and death, a thriving healthcare system or a declining one, and an economically prosperous society or one burdened by debt. Addressing this problem by increasing the representation of physicians, nurses, and allied health professionals from diverse backgrounds is a significant and worthwhile investment in creating a more just, equitable, and effective healthcare system.

A more diverse medical workforce yields numerous benefits, including enhanced communication, a more compassionate approach to patient care, and improved health outcomes. Patients from diverse backgrounds may feel more at ease discussing their medical history, symptoms, and concerns with physicians they assume understand their cultural values and beliefs. Additionally, physicians from diverse backgrounds may better understand the social determinants of health that influence their patients' well-being. This holistic perspective enables them to provide more accurate diagnoses and develop better-tailored treatment plans. By embracing diversity in healthcare, we create an environment where patients feel heard, understood, and respected, leading to positive experiences and better health for all.

Access to Care

Access to care is a complex problem that plagues our nation and is a crucial driver of healthcare disparities. Under this umbrella, various obstacles contribute to the challenge, including affordability, language barriers, the stigma associated with certain conditions, and, notably, the location of healthcare providers. While each factor is essential, let's focus on provider distribution and availability issues, as it directly impacts underserved areas.

If every medical school personal statement translated into reality, our healthcare system would be in great shape. However, the romantic aspirations expressed in these statements often face the harsh realities of life. Students and young clinicians, who are the lifeblood of our healthcare workforce, enter the field with enthusiasm and a desire to solve problems. Over the years, I have read numerous personal statements filled with hope and promises to transform the field. Many express a commitment to practicing in underserved areas. However, as these students transition into young doctors, life's challenges and demands often lead them to adjust their priorities. Medical school loans, families, and retirement needs contribute to young doctors not practicing in poorly resourced areas. Consequently, our nation's underserved areas suffer from inadequate healthcare resources.

I am fortunate to know an exceptional doctor who serves as a shining example of what it means to work in low-resource communities. My wife, my girlfriend then, made it clear from the beginning of her medical journey that she wanted to work in an underserved community. Her goal was to provide preventative services to the most vulnerable populations, and when she completed her training, that's precisely what she did. She deliberately sought employment at a federally qualified health center catering to underserved populations.

When I asked her why she chose this particular setting, her response was insightful and inspiring. She explained, "I felt comfortable caring for this population because I trained at Meharry, a Historically Black College, and University that highly values care for the underserved. I received training with a specific emphasis on this population. And my shared cultural background allowed me to relate to these patients I genuinely care about." Her response left me amazed because it perfectly encapsulated several crucial points that are essential to address.

First, her training at a Historically Black College and University gave her a foundation to feel comfortable and confident in caring for underserved patients. The institution emphasized serving this population and equipped her with the necessary skills and knowledge. Second, her shared cultural background with these patients allowed her to establish a deeper connection and understanding of their unique needs and challenges. This shared background enabled her to provide more personal and empathetic care.

I am incredibly proud of my wife and her contributions to improving healthcare access for underserved populations. However, she is not alone in this fight. A study conducted by Marrast et al. in 2014 revealed a crucial finding related to access to care. The research indicated that nonwhite physicians were responsible for providing over 50% of minority patients' usual care and over 70% of non-English speaking patients' usual care. This statistic is eye-opening and underscores the vital role that minority physicians play in delivering healthcare to underserved communities. It highlights their significant contributions to addressing health disparities, particularly those facing language barriers when accessing healthcare services.

The Marrast study's findings have far-reaching implications beyond numbers and data. Minority physicians, who tend to work in areas with limited access to healthcare, play a crucial role in our medical system. Their understanding of diverse cultures and languages enables them to communicate effectively and truly grasp the needs of their diverse patients. By bridging the gaps in culture and language, these doctors create an atmosphere of trust and mutual understanding, leading to better communication between patients and healthcare providers.

This significantly impacts patient satisfaction, as patients feel listened to, valued, and understood. Meeting patients where they are is essential to improving outcomes, and that's precisely what these physicians practicing in underserved areas are doing.

Increased Cultural Competency

"The more we learn about other cultures, the more we realize how interconnected and interdependent we truly are." - Mae Jemison

Here's a multiple-choice question: Which of the three scenarios would allow you to learn the most about a particular culture?

(A) Reading a book about that culture

(B) Spending meaningful time with people from that culture

(C) Living in that culture

Most people would select the answer "C," and I agree.

The United States is going through a significant demographic shift, where racial and ethnic groups once seen as minorities are projected to become the majority by 2045, according to the US Census Bureau. This demographic change raises an important question: If the medical workforce does not reflect this diversity, will we be able to provide exceptional healthcare to this increasingly diverse population? The urgency to address this question arises from the understanding that it is not only access to care, but access to culturally competent care that is vital in reducing health disparities and ensuring better healthcare for everyone, regardless of their background.

Increasing diversity within the healthcare workforce in proportion to the changing population is crucial to meet the evolving needs of the people. I must reiterate that it's not just about having diverse representation but about delivering culturally competent care to keep our nation's constituents healthy. Culturally competent healthcare considers diverse patient populations' unique values, beliefs, and practices. When patients receive care from healthcare providers who share their cultural background or have received training to understand and respect their cultural nuances, culturally competent care can be delivered at its highest level.

When considering the multiple-choice question, it becomes evident that living in a particular culture offers the most comprehensive and immersive learning experience. It allows individuals to fully immerse themselves in that culture's customs, traditions, and daily life, providing a deeper understanding of its nuances and complexities. Living in a culture exposes individuals to various experiences, interactions, and observations contributing to a more comprehensive perspective and knowledge base.

The ultimate goal of the healthcare system in the United States is to ensure the provision of high-quality care for all individuals and promote a healthy nation. Achieving this goal requires recognizing and addressing the unique needs and perspectives of people from diverse cultures. Cultural competency plays a vital role in this process. It involves understanding the norms and values of different communities and developing the skills and capacity to effectively navigate and engage with individuals from these cultures. In a country as diverse as the United States, cultural competence is essential to achieving optimal healthcare outcomes and ensuring equitable care.

While living in a culture is the most effective way to develop cultural competence, it is not always feasible or practical for healthcare professionals in training to relocate. In such cases, the next best option is actively engaging with individuals from different cultures. By building meaningful relationships and spending time with people from diverse backgrounds, healthcare professionals can gain firsthand knowledge and understanding of cultural norms, practices, and beliefs relevant to their patients. This vicarious experiential learning contributes to their ability to deliver effective patient-centered care, considering the cultural factors influencing health beliefs, behaviors, and treatment preferences.

In our documentary film, "Black Men in White Coats," Dr. Valerie Montgomery-Rice highlights a significant issue within medical schools in the United States—that is, some medical schools produce graduating classes without representation of certain racial or ethnic groups. This lack of diversity can be considered an educational, cultural deficiency and has real societal implications. It reflects a gap in cultural understanding and may result in healthcare professionals who are not adequately prepared to meet the needs of diverse patient populations. Including individuals from various backgrounds in medical education is crucial to foster a learning environment with cultural competency that can move us towards equitable healthcare for all. Simply put, we can grow by intimately interacting with individuals with different backgrounds than our own.

I'm reminded of my freshman year in college. As a black male, just one month into being 18 years old, I found myself sharing a room with a white male from St. Charles, Missouri. It was evident from the start that we were two very different people. We had different interests and different backgrounds. However, the year we spent as roommates was an extraordinary and transformative experience for both of us.

As we got to know each other deeper, we formed a strong bond and became great friends. Our friendship extended beyond the confines of our room, as my friends became his friends and vice versa. Through this interconnectedness, we had the opportunity to immerse ourselves in each other's cultures and expand our horizons. For instance, I discovered new music that resonated with him while he embraced and appreciated the music that was meaningful to me. I can vividly recall waking up to the melodic tones of his Bob Marley alarm, singing, "Is this love... Is this love... Is this love... Is this love that I'm feeling?" This shared experience of cultural exchange left an indelible mark on our college journey, enriching our lives and fostering personal growth.

The absence of diversity within the medical school classroom or healthcare settings has far-reaching implications. It deprives healthcare providers of the opportunity to develop invaluable cultural knowledge and skills for delivering effective patient care. Without exposure to diverse perspectives and experiences, it becomes challenging for healthcare professionals to provide culturally competent care to patients from various backgrounds. It is through diversity in the workforce that providers can learn from their colleagues and broaden their understanding of different cultures. While reading textbooks and attending lectures certainly have merits, they can only provide a limited understanding of cultural nuances. True cultural competency is nurtured through genuine engagement with individuals from diverse backgrounds. It is through these interactions and relationships that healthcare providers gain a deeper appreciation of their patient's unique values, beliefs, and needs.

Cultural competency mandates diving headfirst into the vibrant tapestry of human experiences, where diversity becomes a spark that fuels personal and professional growth. As we build a diverse healthcare workforce, we are creating a space that encourages sharing ideas, challenges old ways of thinking, and fosters a deep understanding of different cultures. Healthcare professionals aren't just there to dish out medical treatments; they also stand up for their patients' rights. Cultural competency is a secret weapon ensuring everyone gets optimal care. When we embrace diversity in medical education and healthcare settings, we give healthcare providers the superpowers they need to navigate the intricate dance between culture, health, and well-being.

Contributions to Research and Innovation

"Something the Lord Made", is one of my favorite movies. The plot revolves around the life of Dr. Vivien Thomas, brilliantly portrayed by the hip-hop artist Mos Def. Dr. Thomas, a black surgical technician, made remarkable contributions to cardiac surgery. The film chronicled his journey in the 1940s when he was hired by Dr. Alfred Blalock, a renowned white surgeon at Johns Hopkins University. Their collaboration focused on researching the treatment of blue baby syndrome, a condition characterized by cardiopulmonary anomalies causing insufficient oxygen in the blood, resulting in a bluish skin color.

Working side by side, Blalock and Thomas embarked on developing a groundbreaking surgical technique to correct the condition. Their innovation involved connecting the aorta and pulmonary artery, enabling a greater flow of oxygen-rich blood to reach the lungs. One of the most poignant scenes in the movie takes place in the operating room. Dr. Blalock, surrounded by a packed auditorium of eager doctors, is preparing to perform the procedure for the first time on a human patient. However, overcome with unease, Blalock abruptly exits the operating room and urgently requests the presence of Thomas. Faced with resistance from the staff because Thomas is black, Blalock emphatically takes matters into his own hands and forcefully pages Thomas over the hospital's sound system.

"Vivien Thomas. Paging Vivien Thomas. You're wanted in the OR right now. Come on the run, do you hear. This is Blalock!"

To the astonishment of everyone present, Blalock and Thomas re-enter the operating room together. With Thomas providing guidance, they successfully carry out the surgery, defying expectations and showcasing the power of their partnership. This pivotal moment exemplifies the immense trust and respect Blalock had for Thomas, recognizing his expertise and invaluable contributions to their shared mission.

Dr. Vivien Thomas's story is one of unwavering dedication, purpose, and triumph over adversity. Despite being told that his aspirations were unattainable, he channeled his determination into working harder than anyone else and making a lasting impact on society. His journey serves as an inspiration not only for individuals facing similar challenges but for all those who strive to overcome barriers and leave a meaningful legacy. Dr. Thomas's story resonates deeply as a testament to the power of perseverance and the ability to defy expectations to pursue one's dreams.

One could hear this story and simply think that his race had nothing to do with the operation's success. If that is your conclusion, you're entirely missing the point. The message is: you never know what contributions someone can make if you exclude them and prohibit them from sharing their gifts and talents. Dr. Thomas's upbringing and years of chasing dreams in search of a better life honed a "no quit" mentality in him.

That exact mentality made it possible for him to walk alongside Dr. Blalock as they made one of the most monumental advancements in the medical field.

Diversity is vital to innovation and advancements in research. Without it, we will likely miss a wealth of perspectives, ideas, and talents that could have made all the difference. When we bring together people from different backgrounds, we tap into various experiences, knowledge, and skills to help us see problems and solutions in new and exciting ways.

A striking example of diversity in action is the Human Genome Project. This ambitious project aimed to sequence the entire human genome, requiring massive collaboration and coordination. Scientists from around the world came together to work on this project, and their diverse perspectives and expertise allowed them to tackle some of the most complex challenges of the project. For example, the project had to deal with the challenge of genetic variation - people from different regions and ethnicities have different genetic variations, which made it difficult to create a reference genome. However, the team's diversity allowed them to identify and incorporate these variations into the reference genome. This led to a more accurate and comprehensive genome sequence, which has been critical in advancing our understanding of human genetics.

Another example of diversity in action is the cochlear implant development, a device that can restore hearing in people with severe hearing loss. The cochlear implant was developed by a team of scientists and engineers who brought together expertise from multiple disciplines, including medicine, biology, engineering, and psychology. The team also included people from diverse backgrounds, including individuals with hearing loss, who provided invaluable insights into the challenges and opportunities of the technology. The team's diversity allowed them to identify and overcome technical challenges, such as how to transmit signals from the implant to the brain, and cultural challenges, such as how to design a socially acceptable device accessible to people from diverse backgrounds.

A more recent example of diversity's contribution to innovation in healthcare is Dr. Kizzmekia Corbett. Her contributions have been invaluable, especially during the COVID-19 pandemic. As one of the lead scientists in developing the Moderna COVID-19 vaccine, she played a crucial role in the fight against the pandemic. Dr. Corbett's groundbreaking work in vaccine development highlights the importance of diversity in STEM fields.

In a personal story shared by Dr. Corbett, she highlights how diversity is essential to the success of any team, including those in healthcare and science. During a therapy session, she expressed frustration that she felt she was doing most of the work in planning family gatherings while her siblings were not contributing meaningfully. Her therapist challenged her to write down one thing each of her siblings did to contribute to the gatherings. In doing this activity, Dr. Corbett realized how each of her siblings played a crucial role in making the gatherings successful and how important their diverse contributions were.

This personal experience helped Dr. Corbett understand the significance of diverse contributions to science and healthcare. In her words, "Diversity in science is not just a matter of checking a box or filling a quota. It's about building the best teams with the most creative ideas and the broadest perspectives." By including individuals from diverse backgrounds, experiences, and perspectives, teams are more likely to produce innovative and practical solutions to complex problems.

Dr. Corbett's work and her insights on diversity have paved the way for greater inclusion in STEM fields, and her example serves as a reminder of the importance of recognizing and valuing diverse contributions. As we continue to address the challenges in healthcare and science, we must strive for greater diversity and inclusion in all aspects of research and innovation.

It's worth emphasizing that the examples cited are just the tip of the iceberg. Healthcare professionals from diverse backgrounds make daily critical contributions, bringing unique experiences and perspectives that enrich the medical field and benefit society. Each individual's story adds to the collective narrative, forging a path toward greater understanding and progress. As such, every voice and perspective is vital; without them, we risk falling short of our full potential.

Changing the Narrative

When my son Jace, a bright and curious seven-year-old, dropped a bombshell during a casual dinner conversation, it made me realize the power of representation on a child's dreams. We were talking about presidents, and I casually mentioned that maybe one day he could be the president of the United States. In response, Jace hit me with a statement that left me speechless. He said, "Daddy, I can't be president."

Surprised, I asked him why not. And what he said next hit me hard. "Because I'm black, Daddy."

It was a wake-up call, showing me how deeply ingrained societal biases can impact a child's beliefs about what he or she can achieve. But here's the thing: if you asked Jace or his siblings if they could become doctors, they would confidently shout,

"Yes!" It's not because they're dying to become doctors, but because they see me, their dad, practicing medicine daily. And it doesn't stop there—my wife is also a doctor. So, for them, seeing doctors in the family is normal. And because of that, becoming one is an ordinary achievement to them.

It's interesting to note that even though Jace lived through Barack Obama's presidency, he didn't fully grasp the significance of having a black president. All he remembered were the lessons about George Washington and Abraham Lincoln. To him, being president wasn't something a black person could do—it wasn't part of his reality.

Jace's innocent remark made me realize how vital it is for children to see people who look like them in positions of power and influence. It's about breaking down barriers and providing diverse role models. When kids see leaders who share their backgrounds, it opens up a world of possibilities. It gives them the confidence to dream big, knowing their race or ethnicity doesn't limit their potential.

Jace's words serve as a reminder that representation matters. It's not just a buzzword; it's a powerful force that shapes a child's beliefs about what they can achieve. By diversifying leadership positions and giving marginalized communities a seat at the table, we empower children like my son to believe in themselves and chase their dreams without limitations. This, in turn, can lead to a more prosperous nation.

Narratives hold immense power in shaping our beliefs, expectations, and how we see ourselves, especially for young people. The media we consume, whether books, movies, or TV shows, significantly influence our choices and dreams. That's why diversity in healthcare is so significant—it's about showcasing excellence and inspiring the next generation.

There's a quote that recently caught fire after we released our "Black Men In White Coats" documentary. "You can't be what you can't see." People started attributing this quote to me, but I must give credit where it's due. As far as I can tell from a quick online search, this powerful statement was coined by the children's rights activist Marian Wright Edelman. While I admit I'm unfamiliar with her work, the quote nonetheless remains profound. It highlights the often-underestimated importance of diversity in the medical field and its impact on shaping the aspirations of future generations.

Think about Dr. Heathcliff Huxtable, the fictional character from the hit series, The Cosby Show. For many black men of my generation, this character represented a gold standard, someone to look up to. Dr. Huxtable's success as a doctor, his beautiful wife, and his comfortable lifestyle became a new narrative, showing black children what they could achieve in their own lives, even though the show was not meant to have a medical focus.

In today's world, social media has become a powerful tool for actual doctors to shape the narrative and inspire young people. This is where diversity in healthcare truly shines. When young individuals from all backgrounds see medical professionals who look like them succeeding and making a difference, it changes their expectations and opens new possibilities. By showcasing diverse medical professionals on social media, we can rewrite the story, inspiring more young people to pursue a career in medicine and creating a more inclusive and diverse healthcare system.

Increased Life Expectancy.

Diversity is not only a matter of representation and inclusivity; it also has a measurable impact on life expectancy. A study by Snyder et al., titled "Black Representation in the Primary Care Physician Workforce and Its Association With Population Life Expectancy and Mortality Rates in the US," delves into the complex relationship between the racial composition of primary care physicians and health outcomes. This groundbreaking research reveals a previously unrecognized connection that holds immense potential for approaching equity in healthcare and improving the well-being of communities.

To unravel this relationship, the study meticulously analyzed data from diverse communities across the United States, examining the racial composition of the primary care physician workforce and its correlation with population-level health outcomes. The results of the study are truly astounding. The investigators found that as the percentage of Black primary care doctors increased within a community, the life expectancy of its residents also significantly rose. This finding underscores the transformative power of diverse primary care physicians who can address marginalized communities' unique healthcare needs and experiences.

The implications of this study are profound and far-reaching. It transcends the boundaries of diversity initiatives and highlights the direct impact that representation in the medical field can have on public health. Putting the results of Synder's study into practice, the logical step would be to actively increase racial and ethnic diversity in the primary care workforce. It is a step towards ensuring that all Americans have the opportunity for a longer and healthier life.

Chapter 4

RACISM IN MEDICINE

"DALE, PLEASE GO SEE our patient in exam room 3. I'll be there in a few minutes. Just get started with the history and physical."

I remember the moment as if it were yesterday. It was one of my first experiences as a third-year medical student, and I was excited to be out of the classroom and interacting with real patients. My patient was an older white man, likely in his late seventies to mid eighties. I eagerly rushed to the patient's room to obtain a comprehensive history and conduct a thorough physical exam on my patient. Unfortunately, the encounter didn't go as expected.

"Good morning. My name is Dale Okorodudu. I'm the medical student working with your doctor today, and she'll be joining us shortly."

I barely got the last word out before the patient asked, "Your name is what?"

"Dale Okorodudu," I replied.

"Oh boy, honey," he said, looking at his daughter with concern and then turning back to me. "What kind of name is that? You're not from around here, are you? You from Africa or something?"

I could feel my frustration building, but I held it in. "Yes, sir, I'm from Nigeria, but I was raised here in America."

He smirked. "Nigeria. Do you know what you're doing? Do they even have doctors there?"

Slightly frustrated, I spoke up to defend myself in what I believed was a polite manner. "Sir, I was raised here in America, and I am a medical student right here. My African heritage has nothing to do with my ability to care for you."

That wasn't enough for him. His unease appeared to grow, and I was scared about where this was going. Fortunately, my supervising clinician entered the room soon after and witnessed his racist shenanigans and disdain toward me. Without hesitation, she chewed him out like a pack of gum. She let him know that his behavior was unacceptable and in no shape or fashion would she tolerate it. Among the many memories throughout my career thus far, this remains one of the most memorable. She didn't have to defend me the way she did, but she chose to. That gave me hope in our medical system.

I wish I could say that was the only time something like that happened to me, but it's not. Even now, as a fully licensed triple board-certified attending physician, I encounter similar situations. Just last week, a patient asked me if I was the doctor in charge. After I replied with an affirmative, he rolled his eyes in disappointment, then looked away with a groan saying, "Oh great." Mind you, he was just meeting me for the first time and didn't know who I was. He had nothing to judge me on except my appearance.

What do these two examples demonstrate? That I don't look like a doctor, at least the image of what many Americans expect a doctor to look like. Although the two previous examples involved white male patients, I have encountered similar scenarios with black patients as well. I recall a patient who mistook me for a member of the hospital transport team, showing more interest in where I was taking him than in my role as the physician responsible for his medical care. I've had a black patient's daughter look at me and then ask when the head doctor was coming to see her dad. Surprise... it's me!

Reflecting on these instances, I'm challenged to not blame the patients and their families. These experiences have taught me that patients' mistrust, uncertainty, and discomfort towards me as their physician may not stem from intentional discrimination but rather from ingrained stereotypes that they have been conditioned to believe. As a black physician with a Nigerian name, I'm not who they expect to be their doctor. I don't fit the description. Understandably, my looks can make patients hesitant to trust me or even want me to be their doctor. Regardless, that doesn't make it right.

It's frustrating, to say the least. As a physician, my job is to provide the best care possible to my patients. But when I walk into a room and see the surprise or concern on a patient's face, it provides an extra layer to caring for them. Keep in mind, many of these patients are already medically complex. Now, not only do I need to figure out their medical pathologies, but I also have to determine if they trust me to care for them and will adhere to my management plans. It's a reminder that, despite all my training and education, there are still people out there who will judge me based on the color of my skin or the sound of my name. It's a reminder that racism is a real thing in medicine that has real implications for patient care.

I know all too well the sting of being stereotyped and the frustration of patients doubting my clinical abilities before even meeting me. It's a feeling of being dismissed and overlooked, and it's disheartening. But what hurts even more, is when my colleagues and trainees undermine my position. At times, I've questioned my sensitivity to this topic. I've wondered if I'm overreacting or if other doctors with various backgrounds experience the same perceived lack of respect. But it's the little things that add up: staff calling me by my first name while addressing everyone else as "Doctor," or a colleague seeking guidance from a pulmonary doctor and directing their questions to my trainee, even though I'm the one providing all the answers and look significantly older.

These microaggressions may seem small, but they take a toll over time. Constantly, I find myself analyzing these situations and wondering if I should speak up or let it go. And by no means do I believe I'm alone in this. I know that if it's happening to me, it's likely happening to other underrepresented physicians, too. Ultimately, this results in an extra level of stress added to an already challenging job. It demands a higher level of performance as I strive to be respected for the craft I've worked hard to master. It's a greater responsibility, knowing that the next black physician may face the same disrespect, and therefore it's up to me to change the narrative for them. And while I've considered changing my style to project a more dominant persona, I know that won't solve the underlying problem.

Reflecting on these experiences, I am reminded of a valuable lesson I learned in medical school. Interestingly enough, this specific lesson I'm referring to didn't come from my school (although I must mention that I absolutely loved my medical school). As previously stated, my wife was a student at Meharry Medical College, which is a Historically Black College and University (HBCU). I spent much of my free time on their campus during my fourth year of medical school. In fact, her classmates often mistook me for a fellow student, and to this day, I am sometimes invited to their reunions and other events. Often, I find myself reminding them that it was my wife who was the Meharry graduate, not me.

During their capstone class held just before their graduation, I learned this lesson from Dr. Wayne Riley, who was the president of the academic system at the time. Dr. Riley shared his personal story and the struggles he overcame to achieve his position, emphasizing that every student earning a Medical Degree from Meharry should never forget that their MD is worth as much as anyone else's MD. He implored the students to be proud of their accomplishments and to never allow anyone to demean them because of their appearance or where they obtained their degrees. This line of thought continues to be a great source of strength as I progress through my career.

Atrocities of the Past

"Those who do not know the past are bound to repeat it." – George Santayana

This sentiment, among others, drives me to raise a generation of leaders in medicine from diverse backgrounds. At times, I think life would be easier if I simply relieved myself of these efforts and just took care of my patients. No added work; just be an exceptional doctor. However, when I consider the history of medicine in America and the heinous acts committed against those in disadvantaged positions, I am frightened for the future should we not achieve a more diverse physician workforce. Let's consider a few medical atrocities of the past.

The Tuskegee Syphilis Study

The Tuskegee Syphilis Study remains a harrowing reminder of the grave consequences that arise when scientific exploration is unchecked by ethical considerations. The study, conducted by the US Public Health Service for four decades, targeted African American men who were already marginalized by society. Despite being promised free healthcare, the study participants were deliberately denied treatment for syphilis, even when a cure had become widely available. According to one of the study's researchers, Dr. Taliaferro Clark, "The men's status did not warrant ethical debate. They were subjects, not patients; clinical material, not sick people."

This inhumane study was finally halted in 1972 when it was exposed by the media, causing a national uproar. When asked about the project, Dr. Sidney Olansky, who served as the study's assistant director, reportedly said, "The men were expendable... They were just a means to an end."

The Tuskegee Syphilis Study is a stark reminder of the dangers of unchecked medical experimentation on vulnerable populations. Its disregard for ethical principles and the dignity of human life highlights the importance of diversity in healthcare and the need for representation and advocacy for marginalized groups. As Dr. Vanessa Gamble, a scholar of medical ethics and the granddaughter of a participant, noted, "The study was a result of systemic racism and white supremacy... It's important that we recognize that the medical profession, like any other profession, can be used as a tool of oppression and subjugation."

Forced Sterilization

The forced sterilization of women of color in America is a shameful chapter in our country's history. This practice, which was part of the eugenics movement, aimed to control the reproductive rights of people deemed "unfit" to reproduce, including those with mental illness or disabilities. Unfortunately, this policy disproportionately targeted women of color, who were often coerced or forced into sterilization procedures.

One of the most notorious cases of forced sterilization was that of Elaine Riddick, an African American woman who was sterilized without her consent at the age of 14 while she was in a North Carolina state home for "delinquent" girls. She later recalled, "They told me I was going to have stitches, and when I woke up, I was sterilized." Riddick's story is just one of many that shed light on the devastating impact of forced sterilization on women of color.

Henrietta Lacks

In the mid-twentieth century, prisoners were often used as guinea pigs for medical experimentation. The most infamous example of this is the case of Henrietta Lacks, a Black woman whose cancer cells were harvested without her knowledge or consent and used for scientific research. Lacks' cells, which were immortal and able to reproduce indefinitely, have since been used to develop numerous medical treatments.

Lacks' family was never informed about the use of her cells for medical experimentation, and for decades they had no idea that her cells were being used in labs around the world. In her book "The Immortal Life of Henrietta Lacks," author Rebecca Skloot details the family's discovery of the use of Lacks' cells and their subsequent fight for recognition and compensation.

As Lacks' daughter, Deborah, recounted, "My mother was used in medical experiments without her knowledge or consent...and her family was never told. They took her cells and didn't even ask." The exploitation of Lacks' cells without her consent raises essential questions about medical ethics and informed consent. It also highlights the long-standing issue of medical exploitation and abuse of marginalized communities.

These are just a few examples of the many medical atrocities committed against minorities throughout American history. These actions have caused significant harm and lingering mistrust within these communities. Reflecting on them, the question that plagues my mind is rooted in the very foundation of our history: how and why did these ghastly medical atrocities come to be?

The answer is complex, but a crucial factor is the glaring absence of diversity in the field. When a moral voice of authority was desperately needed to intervene and condemn these sins, there was no one in power to do so. No one could wholeheartedly relate to the victims and inspire the courage to declare with conviction, "No! This is wrong. Don't do it." These unforgettable offenses were committed in part as a direct result of the lack of representation in healthcare. Let's remember our history and make the necessary adjustments to ensure these acts of evil never happen again.

Systemic Racism

Consider this hypothetical situation. You play the lottery and win $1 billion dollars, but there's a catch: you can't spend any of the money on yourself and have to give it away. Now, I'd like you to think of the first five people you'd give money to. Now think of the following five. Now the next five. And one more time, think of the next five.

I'm willing to bet that for most of you, the first five to ten were either family members or very close friends. The following five to ten likely aren't quite as close to you but are still family, friends, or acquaintances. There's nothing wrong with that, and it's probably what I'd do as well. It's human nature. It's also the foundation for systemic racism.

At its core, systemic racism refers to the ways in which society is structured that disproportionately benefit some groups while disadvantaging others. It is an insidious force that has shaped our institutions and systems in ways that many of us do not even realize. But to understand systemic racism, we must first understand how our natural biases play a role in its creation.

It is thought that our natural biases are programmed into us from a young age. They are a product of our upbringing, our culture, and our personal experiences. These biases inform our decision-making processes, influencing who we trust, who we empathize with, and who we choose to help. It is this last factor that is particularly important when it comes to understanding systemic racism.

When we think about the first few people we would give money to in the lottery example, we are likely to think about those closest to us. For example, the first person I'd give to is my wife. Our natural biases compel us to help those we know and love. They also compel us to help those that are more likely to help us. Again, there's nothing inherently wrong with this; it's a natural part of being human. However, when we extend this logic to the broader society, it can have unintended consequences.

If we only, or primarily, help those closest to us, we are creating a system that benefits some while leaving others behind. For example, if we only help our family members and close friends get jobs or receive promotions, we are effectively excluding others who may be equally qualified. Over time, this exclusion can compound, leading to entire groups of people being disenfranchised.

This is how systemic racism develops. It's not necessarily intentional or malicious, but it is real and is the result of our natural biases playing out on a larger scale. In order to combat systemic racism, we must first recognize these biases and work to overcome them, at least to some extent. We must be intentional in our efforts to help those who are different from us, to empathize with their experiences, and to ensure that our actions do not perpetuate systemic inequalities.

Considering this, I'm reminded of the story of the Good Samaritan, a well-known and frequently referenced parable from the Bible. It is a tale of kindness and compassion that illustrates the importance of helping others in need. However, the story also has a deeper meaning that speaks to the issue of systemic racism.

The parable begins with a man traveling from Jericho to Jerusalem. Along the way, he is attacked by robbers and left for dead. As he lies on the ground, two men pass by a priest and a Levite. Both of these individuals were highly respected members of the Jewish community and would have been expected to help the injured man. However, they both continue on their way without offering any assistance.

It is not until a Samaritan man comes along that the injured traveler receives help. The traditional teaching of this parable explains that Samaritans were viewed as outsiders and sometimes had friction with the Jewish community. Yet, it is the Samaritan who stops to help the man, taking him to an inn, caring for him, and even leaving money with the innkeeper to ensure that he is well taken care of.

Jesus tells this parable in response to a question about who one's neighbor is. By using a Samaritan as the hero of the story, Jesus challenges his listeners to reconsider their preconceived notions about who is worthy of help and compassion. He is urging them to expand their definition of "neighbor" to include those who may be different from themselves and consider all in need.

To fully comprehend the gravity of this parable, it is vital to recognize that it was delivered from a Jewish perspective. As I understand, throughout history, there has been a palpable tension between Jewish and Samaritan societies, adding depth to the story's underlying message. Despite the injured man being presumed Jewish, those who would be expected to provide assistance, such as the priest and the Levite, chose to ignore his plight. It is the Samaritan, who would have been viewed as an outsider and less likely to offer aid, that goes out of his way to help the traveler. The Samaritan, rather than the man's own kin or religious leaders, exemplified the true meaning of being a neighbor.

One of the most bothersome aspects of systemic racism is the way in which it operates on a subconscious level. Our natural biases and prejudices can cause us to make assumptions about others and mistreat them, even if we do not intend to do so. This is what makes the story of the Good Samaritan so powerful - it shows that it is possible to work against these biases and do what is right, even if it requires inconveniencing ourselves.

In the context of healthcare, the parable of the Good Samaritan carries profound significance. Just as the injured man in the story encountered unexpected assistance from an outsider, we, too, must embrace diversity and inclusivity within the healthcare system. By challenging our subconscious biases and embracing a broader definition of who deserves care and compassion, we can ensure that no patient is overlooked or marginalized. Just as the Samaritan went out of his way to help the traveler, we must be willing to go beyond the status quo and actively work to dismantle systemic racism and inequalities in healthcare. In doing so, we can truly exemplify the essence of being a neighbor and build a healthcare system that offers equal care and opportunity for all, regardless of their background or identity.

Chapter 5

EMPOWERING
COMMUNITIES

In our documentary, "Black Men In White Coats," my older brother Daniel and I engage in a lively debate on the question of who bears the responsibility for increasing the number of black men in medicine. Daniel argues that the community holds the primary responsibility, while I contend that medical schools should take the lead in addressing this issue.

When we sit on Q&A panels, people love asking us this question. It's as if they want to see the argument play out just for the sake of entertainment. And while we may have exaggerated the film's scene just a little to make it more interesting, the truth of the matter is both perspectives are valid.

Unleashed

The most significant barriers to eliminate are the ones within a child's mind. Daniel, who is an endocrinologist, once told me about an encounter he had while in clinic.

He was seeing a patient who brought her son along for the doctor's visit. Wanting to inspire the youth, my brother asked, "What do you want to be when you grow up?"

The elementary-age child shrugged his shoulders, uncertain as many kids are.

Daniel continued, "How about becoming a doctor. That'd be pretty cool, right? What do you think about that?"

As Daniel tells it, before the boy could open his mouth to answer, his mother interrupted and shut that door close.

Laughing, she answered, "Ya right. He can't be a doctor."

Some people are going to read this and immediately criticize this mother. That'd be the wrong thing to do. No progress will be made with that approach. Instead, take a step back and ask why she responded that way? It's likely because that's what she knows. I'm sure she loves her child and wants what's best for him. This mother wasn't trying to shatter her son's opportunities; on the contrary, she was seeking to protect him. It's entirely possible that she didn't want my brother filling her child's head with what she believed to be false hopes and aspirations toward a profession she deemed too challenging to enter.

It's important to note the black community is not monolithic. This example is not meant to be representative of all black families. It's simply an illustration that provides perspective on barriers faced by some, not all, youth in our community. While this example holds true in specific households, it is not by any means a universal notion.

Beyond this mother not wanting to set her son up for failure, we must remember the history of America. Black people have been told for centuries that they can't do certain things. Imagine being a slave and constantly being told you're dumb. Imagine not being allowed to read. Imagine knowing that you have one occupation choice for your entire life, slavery. In this brainwashing process, core beliefs are established that can drown one's view of self. The abolition of slavery may have provided a level of physical freedom; however, it's been said that many former slaves and their descendants carried on with remnants of mental bondage.

In 2013, I met a gentleman by the name of Joel Wiggins. My buddy Darius, traveled down from Durham to Dallas to help Joel move into his new home. Joel was, and is, a well-to-do man who has experienced great success since a young age.

One evening, outside of his mansion, Joel began speaking to me with what I'd consider an anointed authority. Staring deep into my soul, he said, "You don't even see it do you, Dale?"

I stood there, having no idea what he was talking about. We were standing outside of his ginormous house in his circle driveway, and he was yelling at me for the entire neighborhood to see.

He continued. "That's your problem, Dale; you don't realize you have permission to be great."

I wondered if I should jump in my car and speed away. This man, whom I barely knew, thought he could speak to me as if I was a child. Should I stand for this disrespect or give him my two cents about his arrogance to talk to me this way. Then he said something that has stuck with me ever since.

"Dale," he called. "Since you won't give it to yourself, I'm going to give it to you. I give you my permission to be great. You have permission to be great!"

Unleashed! That's how I felt, unleashed. And there was nothing anyone could do from that point on to take that permission from me.

For clarification, I was born in Nigeria and am not of black American slave descent. While I may not share a similar lineage to my wife and other black Americans of slave descent, living in this society since age three, I am also impacted by the current systems in place that can hold back underrepresented individuals. In a sense, I had always felt a bondage of sorts; however, nothing near what those who lived under the oppression of slavery experienced.

Although my parents had always told me I could be anything I wanted to be, something about hearing someone else tell me I had permission to be great was very empowering. It was also enlightening as I saw the impact that simple phrase had on me.

Now, as a nationally sought-after speaker, I travel the country spreading this message. Telling children that they have permission to be great is a means to unleash their minds to consider the most extraordinary things life can offer them.

It's also essential that we hold our youth accountable. Yes, there are many barriers that they will face; however, we must not absolve them of their role in their own success. This is what Joel wanted me to understand. The biblical parable of the talents speaks to this.

In the story, a master goes on a trip and leaves three servants with talents (money) to mind. The first two servants invest their talents and double their worth, while the third servant buries his talent and returns it to the master as is. The master rewards the first two servants for their diligence and initiative but punishes the third servant for his laziness and fearfulness.

Underrepresented populations may face systemic barriers and challenges that make it harder for them to achieve success. However, this does not relieve us of our personal responsibility to take the talents we have been given and use them to the best of our abilities. We must encourage our youth to take ownership of their lives and to strive for excellence in all that they do. Ultimately, they must be accountable for their own success, but as educators, parents, and community members, we, too, have a responsibility to support and empower them along the way.

How to Raise a Doctor

"Train up a child in the way he should go, and when he is old, he will not depart from it." – Proverbs 22:6 KJV

Remember the story I told earlier about my son not believing he could be president? Jace felt that way because he didn't know any black presidents and therefore thought it wasn't an option for him. After that occurrence, we had a detailed talk during which I explained to him that, without a doubt, he could become president. Although society set an expectation for him, as his dad, I overruled that and transformed his belief system. That was my responsibility.

In 2018, I published my first book, How to Raise a Doctor: Wisdom from Parents Who Did It. The book was based on the insight I gained from interviewing over 75 parents of physicians. It's an easy and worthwhile read which I highly recommend. One thing quickly became clear from this book project, parents are the ones who lay the foundation for their children's successes. For the most part, the achievements attained are directly related to parents' level of involvement. If we want to see more diversity in healthcare, we must equip parents to prepare their children for such a career. From my research and interviews, I was able to identify three key elements used by parents to guide their children on their path to becoming doctors. They are as follows.

1) Suggest a career in medicine for your child.

When it comes to encouraging children to consider a career in medicine, it's important for parents to take a gentle and supportive approach. While parents shouldn't force their children into any specific career path, they can undoubtedly suggest medicine as an option for them to consider. By doing so, parents are giving their children the opportunity to explore a career in a field that can be incredibly rewarding and fulfilling. Additionally, when parents suggest medicine as a career to their children, they are providing a level of support and encouragement that can be incredibly valuable. Children who know that their parents approve of their career choices are more likely to feel confident and motivated to pursue their goals. By suggesting medicine as a career, parents are giving their children a gentle nudge in the right direction and providing them with the support they need to succeed.

2) Set high expectations for your child.

Setting high expectations for children is crucial for their success, and it was a common theme among the parents of the doctors in my study. These parents focused on ensuring their children performed to their unique potential instead of just meeting basic standards. This mentality helped to create an environment where success was expected and not just hoped for.

Parents who set high expectations for their children play a critical role in shaping their mindset. This approach helps children develop a growth mindset, which instills the belief that their abilities can be developed through dedication and hard work. As a result, when children set high expectations and achieve them, it provides a significant boost in confidence that motivates them to take on even more significant challenges.

In addition to setting high expectations, parents should be aware of the Law of Least Effort. This psychological principle suggests that people tend to expend the minimal amount of energy needed to accomplish a given task. For example, consider two students in the same literature class with different sets of parental expectations. John's parents are satisfied with a passing grade, while Amber's parents expect her to make straight A's. When the teacher assigns an essay, John spends only ten minutes writing a one-page document while Amber conducts extensive research and writes a detailed but succinct essay. As a result, Amber earns an 'A,' and John earns a 'C.'

Who do you think expended more effort? Likely Amber, of course. What's important to recognize here is the amount of effort is correlated to the set expectations. This is critically important because compounding effort leads to compounding results, and that's how sustained success is achieved in the medical field and beyond. Setting high expectations leads to a higher effort level and, more often than not, better results.

Part of setting high expectations is ensuring the child puts in the work to become successful. Specifically, I'm referring to academic success. I'm going to let you in on my little secret. When speaking on stages nationwide, I focus on organizational accountability. In those settings, I speak from a disparities and systemic barriers perspective. The intent here is to emphasize the importance of leveraging system resources to help those in need. However, when I speak at schools and local community events, I emphasize individual accountability and the hard-to-swallow reality that most people don't care if you're struggling, so you better figure things out fast.

Considering the latter, parents, teachers, and community leaders are responsible for pushing the concept of academic excellence. This, perhaps, is the most consistent way to elevate socioeconomic status in America. Education is the key to opportunity. Whether we like it or not, grades matter. Whether we like it or not, standardized tests matter. Because this is true, we must equip youth from diverse backgrounds to score well on these exams and in the classroom. That means education must be a priority from day one.

It is upon us to enforce standards and expectations for our children to counter the myriad of other challenges they will face throughout their lifetime. We've been given a cheat code for their success, and that cheat code is simple, study harder than everyone else! For every hour children spend playing their sport or performing their art, they should spend a proportional amount of time studying. This is the critical mechanism by which we can increase diversity in all professional fields. When it comes to effort, specifically academic effort, the only disparities are the ones we create for ourselves.

3) Learn about your child's potential career.

Finally, to support their children's successes, the parents in my study took the initiative to learn about the profession themselves. They strove to become their children's primary advisors, providing guidance and support throughout their journeys. In the pre-internet days, I recall how my own parents dedicated time to researching the college process and career paths via books and magazines. Their efforts were not for themselves but to gain knowledge that would enable them to offer informed advice and support to their children. With the vast resources available today, it is even more critical for parents to stay informed and involved in their children's pursuit of medicine.

If we genuinely want to increase diversity in healthcare, we must empower communities, and that means empowering parents. Families form the backbone of societies, and it is crucial that we support and uplift each and every one of them. As an author, it is not enough for me to simply write about the importance of empowering parents in my books. I am committed to putting this belief into action, which is why I ensure that every Black Men In White Coats Youth Summit held across the country includes a workshop focused on empowering parents. By providing parents with the tools and knowledge they need to support their children, we are also empowering the next generation of healthcare professionals. After all, the success of our children is ultimately tied to the success of our communities, and it is up to us to ensure that every child has the opportunity to thrive.

The Classroom

"You are not inferior. Your grades may be, and your school may be. But you can turn that around..." – Joe Clark, Lean on Me

Let's be clear, the lack of diversity among healthcare professionals is directly related to the subpar educational system in many underrepresented minority communities. Many talented young boys and girls from these communities are not given the tools they need to succeed, particularly when it comes to pursuing careers in medicine. The key to addressing this problem is to empower teachers and improve the education system as a whole.

The 1989 film "Lean on Me" is one of my favorites. It's a powerful portrayal of the struggles that underprivileged schools face in their efforts to provide an education to their students. The movie is based on a true story and follows the journey of Joe Clark, a high school principal who takes on the daunting task of turning around an inner-city school in Paterson, New Jersey.

The school is plagued with violence, low test scores, and a lack of discipline among its students. Clark is determined to create a safe and nurturing environment for his students, but he faces resistance from the school board, faculty, and even some of the parents.

I challenge you to watch the film and then make a list of all the barriers you can identify that would hinder the students at Eastside High from becoming medical doctors.

Now imagine this, you're a medical school admissions dean with one spot left in your incoming class, and you're considering two students - Ashley, with a 3.4-grade point average, and Bobby, with a 3.9. At first glance, it might seem like a no-brainer to choose the student with the higher GPA. But in reality, that decision is far from clear-cut.

Grades alone do not tell the whole story of a student's potential to become an exceptional doctor. There are numerous factors that contribute to success in the medical field, and a student's grades are just one piece of the puzzle. Unfortunately, too often, we place an exaggerated emphasis on grades as a measure of intelligence and potential when in reality, they are just one aspect of a student's overall academic profile.

It's essential to recognize that not all students have had access to the same quality of education and resources throughout their academic careers. Students from underserved communities, who often face inadequate funding, understaffed schools, and limited access to educational resources, may struggle to achieve top grades even if they possess exceptional intelligence and potential. As a result, relying solely on grades as a measure of a student's aptitude can lead to a lack of diversity in the medical field and a missed opportunity to cultivate talent from underrepresented communities.

The challenges facing teachers and school systems in providing the best education to underrepresented minority students seem endless. These students often attend schools that are underfunded and understaffed, with inadequate resources to support their academic development. Consider Martin Luther King Jr. Elementary School. This school, located in a predominantly African American neighborhood, has struggled with low academic performance for many years. According to data from the Tennessee Department of Education, only 10.9% of third-grade students at this school scored proficient or advanced on the state's math assessment in the 2019-2020 school year. In addition, only 11.9% of third-grade students scored proficient or advanced on the state's English Language Arts assessment.

The school has faced significant challenges due to a lack of funding and resources. For example, in the 2019-2020 school year, the school had a student-teacher ratio of 18:1, which is higher than the national average of 16:1. The school also had a high teacher turnover rate, with many teachers leaving due to low pay and difficult working conditions. This has resulted in a lack of stability and consistency in the classroom, which can be particularly damaging for students who already face significant challenges outside of school.

The impact of these challenges is significant not only for the students but for the local community as well. MLK Elementary School is located in one of the most impoverished neighborhoods in its state, and many of the students come from low-income families. Without access to quality education, these students are at a significant disadvantage in terms of future academic and career opportunities. This, in turn, can perpetuate the generational cycle of poverty and limited opportunities in the community, one of which may be pursuing professional careers in healthcare.

The Teacher Workforce

Let's take a step back. Thus far, we've been focused on diversity at the end of the pipeline, but it'd make sense to examine diversity at the start of the pipeline to see how that may be a contributing factor. Teacher diversity has been a hot topic in the education system for some time now. According to National Center for Education Statistics data (NCES), approximately 79% of public school teachers in the United States are White, while only 7% are Black and 9% are Hispanic. This lack of diversity among teachers has been shown to harm the academic development of underrepresented minority students. Let's take a moment to examine this.

Stereotypes and biases can significantly impact a student's education. Teachers play a critical role in shaping students' academic experiences, and their beliefs and attitudes can affect their academic achievement. Unfortunately, many teachers may hold negative stereotypes or implicit biases towards certain racial or ethnic groups without realizing it and, in doing so, are hindering their progress.

A 2021 study published in the Journal of Educational Psychology found that teachers who held implicit biases toward Black and Hispanic students negatively impact those students' academic achievement. The study involved a sample of nearly 3,000 teachers across the United States. It assessed their implicit biases toward Black and Hispanic students using a measure known as the Implicit Association Test. The researchers found that teachers who held implicit biases towards these groups were more likely to have lower expectations for their academic performance, provide less instructional support, and give them lower grades than their white peers.

These findings are troubling, as they suggest that implicit biases among teachers can contribute to educational disparities and perpetuate systemic racism within the education system. For example, minority students face disproportionate disciplinary action in schools, contributing to a myriad of downstream issues. According to data from the U.S. Department of Education, Black students are three times more likely to be suspended or expelled than white students. This discrepancy has been attributed to the racial biases held by teachers and administrators, which can lead to disproportionate punishment for students of color.

I myself was subject to such disciplinary disparities. I recall having a play fight with a friend when I was in the sixth grade. He and I had known each other for several years and were simply goofing off. Our teacher, I'll call her Mrs. C, had stepped out of the room for a short while. When she returned, she found us in the middle of our WWF royal rumble wrestling match. Her interpretation of the incident was that I was beating up a classmate, and serious disciplinary action was to follow.

I had multiple issues with that same teacher earlier in the year, and I was concerned this may be the last straw. Mind you, I was a pretty "good" kid. Sure, I did the usual pre-teen boy stuff, but I wasn't doing anything that would warrant suspension or being expelled. Finally, it seemed this would be the breaking point where one of those two things would happen.

Thankfully I had very present parents in my life who trusted and believed their child. Papa came to the school and defended his son. The teacher made all sorts of false accusations, including claiming I was a thief who stole candy from other students. My dad knew that was not my character and I wouldn't do such things. In the end, everything was sorted out, and somehow Papa even got Mrs. C to apologize to me.

I think back to that situation and ask myself, what about those students who don't have parents like mine? What would have happened to me if Papa wasn't there? Would I have gotten suspended or expelled? Would I have been labeled a "trouble-maker" student like many other underserving students?

When students are disciplined more than their counterparts at school, the results can be drastic, hindering a child's ultimate level of personal and professional achievement. This can lead to a negative cycle with lasting effects. The fourth-grade failure syndrome is an example of this phenomenon, where students who do not meet grade-level benchmarks in fourth grade are more likely to fall behind in later grades and not graduate high school. This is especially true for minority students who are disciplined at higher rates. In fact, a study conducted by the Civil Rights Project at UCLA found that students who had been suspended or expelled were more likely to be held back a grade, drop out of school, and ultimately have lower academic achievement. So here's my question to you: how do you think this impacts diversity in healthcare?

Diversifying the Teacher Workforce

Okay, now that the problem is clear, let's shift our mindset to solution mode. What would be a simple strategy we could use to address the discipline discrepancy and fourth-grade failure syndrome?

In 2020, a study conducted by the American Educational Research Association found that Black students who had a Black teacher in elementary school were more likely to graduate from high school and attend college. Amazingly, having a Black teacher in elementary school for just one year was associated with a 13% increase in the likelihood of a Black student enrolling in college.

Furthermore, the study also found that having a teacher of the same race positively impacted academic achievement for Black and Hispanic students. Having a Black teacher in elementary school led to a 7% increase in math scores for Black students and a 5% increase for Hispanic students. The same was true for reading scores, where having a Black teacher led to a 10% increase in reading scores for Black students and a 9% increase for Hispanic students.

This study highlights the importance of teacher diversity in the academic success of minority students. The positive impact of having a teacher of the same race is clear, yet the teaching workforce still lacks diversity. Again, only 7% of teachers in the United States are Black, while Black students comprise 15% of the public school student population. This disparity is even greater for Hispanic students, who comprise 28% of the student population but are only represented by 9% of teachers.

Diversifying the educational workforce also brings the benefit of increasing cultural competency among staff. I'm reminded of an instance my peers and I experienced in medical school. Our curriculum was heavily based on a problem-based learning system, so we spent more time-solving cases in a group setting than sitting in lecture halls.

One day, while working on a case, my group opted to take a break. During this time, my group leader, who was a white male psychiatrist, asked if we wanted to hear a joke. Looking for quick entertainment, we said yes. Needless to say, his joke ended up not going so well. He told a story of a boy with Tourette's syndrome who repeatedly said the "N-word." But my professor didn't say the "N-word"; he said the real thing. And he said it over and over and over again. Time and time again, I ask myself how in the world he could have thought that was okay? If he had been surrounded by more diversity, would he have been more culturally sensitive and not used poor taste in telling that joke?

I, directly and indirectly, dealt with that issue for the next two years of my medical school career. In a sense, my black classmates and I became unofficial ambassadors for this issue and others. While other students went to class, studied, and took exams, we did that, but in addition, we spent countless hours working to rectify various diversity issues. Fortunately for us, we still performed well academically, but what about other minority students in similar situations who struggle to manage the standard responsibilities of medical school in addition to these bonus tasks?

The lack of diversity in the teaching workforce contributes to a lack of diversity in the legal profession, medical profession, and more. This not only hinders academic achievement but can also reinforce systemic racism and inequalities in our education system. As a society, we must prioritize increasing teacher diversity to create solutions and advance our nation forward. If we can fix this problem, we'll likely fix many more as a direct result.

Chapter 6

Rethinking
Medical School
Admissions

"**D**R. DALE, WE'RE TRYING our best. We really want to admit more students from minority backgrounds, but there just aren't very many qualified students applying."

I couldn't begin to tell you how many times I've heard this. It's become the age-old, broken record rationale for the lack of diversity in medical school. In basic economics, the supply of qualified, diverse students is limited, while the demand for them is high. This paradigm has created intense competition among medical schools to recruit these students, resulting in a situation where they are all vying for the same students in a small pool of applicants. While I fully understand this predicament, I can't say I agree entirely. Personally, I believe that there are more qualified applicants than we are acknowledging. Furthermore, we must hold medical school admissions committees accountable for doing their due diligence to find these individuals if, in fact, they are out there. In addition, we must also hold each school accountable for the criteria they use to define "qualified."

Let's spend some time dissecting this and rethinking medical school admissions.

The Purpose of Medical Schools

Medical schools exist to produce competent and compassionate physicians who will provide quality healthcare to their patients. To achieve this goal, medical schools provide rigorous academic and clinical training that equips students with the knowledge and skills to diagnose, treat, and prevent diseases. Medical schools also play a critical role in advancing medical research, discovering new treatments, and developing better healthcare systems.

In recent years, however, medical schools are taking on a seemingly more pressing role as they have faced increasing pressure to generate revenue and operate as businesses. The high cost of medical education, the need to attract top faculty and researchers, and the desire to maintain state-of-the-art facilities and equipment have all contributed to the financial focus of medical schools. As a result, medical schools are often evaluated in part based on their financial performance rather than their success in meeting the healthcare needs of society.

This commercialization of medical schools can have several negative consequences. Firstly, it can divert resources away from the core purpose of medical schools, which is to train competent physicians. When financial considerations take precedence over educational objectives, the quality of medical education can suffer. This can lead to a shortage of qualified physicians and poor patient outcomes.

Secondly, commercialization can lead to a focus on profitability over patient care. For example, a medical school may prioritize recruiting high-paying patients or developing lucrative treatments over providing affordable and accessible healthcare to all members of their community. This can contribute to the inequities in healthcare access and outcomes that are already prevalent in many parts of the world.

At the same time, however, we must recognize that for medical education to occur, academic medical centers require adequate funds. Training the next generation of clinicians and serving communities is an extraordinarily immense expense. When a training hospital cannot meet its financial requirements, it may be forced to close. This, in turn, can be devastating for the population it serves.

To stay true to their purpose, medical schools must achieve the proper balance between revenue generation, patient care, and education. For some institutions, this will require a shift in focus from financial performance to social responsibility. Medical schools must embrace their role as institutions that exist to serve society's healthcare needs rather than solely as businesses that must increase profits. The end goal must remain the needs of our patient population.

What Makes a Good Doctor?

Here's a quiz question for you. Which member of the medical team do patients most appreciate? Let's limit this quiz to those holding a medical or osteopathic degree or working towards obtaining one.

For those not accustomed to the traditional team structure, allow me to detail some of the usual players and their roles. Medical students are typically in their third or fourth year of medical school and are learning how to apply their knowledge to clinical situations. They are often responsible for taking the patient's history and performing a physical exam, as well as developing a preliminary diagnosis and treatment plan under the supervision of the attending physician.

Resident physicians, on the other hand, are licensed doctors who have completed medical school and are in the process of completing additional training in a particular specialty. They often have more responsibility for the patient's care and are involved in making clinical decisions under the supervision of the attending physician.

Fellow physicians are doctors who have completed their residency training and are pursuing additional training in a particular subspecialty. They are involved in the patient's care but sometimes may have less direct involvement than the resident physician.

Finally, the attending faculty physician is the senior-most member of the team and is responsible for overseeing the care of all their patients. They provide guidance to the medical students, resident physicians, and fellows. It is the attending doctor who is ultimately responsible for the patient's care.

These medical professionals work together for the sake of the patient. Each member brings their unique knowledge and skill set to the table, ensuring the patient receives a comprehensive and multidisciplinary approach to their care.

Back to our quiz question. Who do you think patients appreciate the most?

Considering the roles listed, the obvious answer would be the attending physician. After all, this individual is the most experienced team member and should also be the most knowledgeable. Would you be surprised if I told you that anecdotally I've seen many instances where the patient prefers discussing their medical issues with the medical student or resident physician? These are the most junior members of the medical team, so what sense does that make? Why is this the case? To understand this, we must investigate what qualities define a good doctor from the patient's perspective.

Several research studies have sought to answer this. In 2020, Borracci et al. surveyed 107 consecutive patients at a community hospital as well as 115 physicians. The authors compared what qualities patients considered meaningful for good doctors to the physicians' opinions. It turns out that patients valued interpersonal social aspects more, whereas doctors focused on aspects of intelligence.

Considering the Borracci study and multiple more with similar findings, it makes sense why patients sometimes value students and younger clinicians more than the supervising faculty doctors. It is because patients value their own insight and opinions. These junior doctors and medical students in training typically spend much more time listening and communicating with the patients. They're at the bedside more. Even when attending doctors are the ones cracking the mystery cases, credit is often given to the ones spending the most time with the patient.

My friend John Boaz once told me about a community in Africa that was being supported by missionaries. Apparently, they were receiving quite a bit of financial support from Americans. The support would have been significant and essential for their sustainability. However, when asked who they were most grateful for, their answer was not the Americans. Many were more grateful to other supporters who hadn't contributed nearly as much financially. The reason was simple: while they appreciated the monetary donations, what they valued more was the time the other missionaries were actually spending with them. They appreciated that these individuals had left the comfort of their own habitats to attend to their needs. To them, that was priceless.

The same is true for our patients in healthcare. Of course, patients value their healthcare providers' diagnostic and therapeutic contributions. However, what many appreciate even more is the medical staff's willingness to spend time with them, listen, and demonstrate care and understanding. It's the interpersonal qualities that patients are looking for. To them, that's a massive part of what makes a good doctor.

Redefining Merit

Merriam-Webster defines merit as a person's qualities, actions, etc., regarded as indicating what the person deserves to receive.

Merit is a complex concept, and when it comes to medical school admissions, it's essential to balance what an individual deserves with what society needs. While academic performance is undoubtedly important, it's not the only factor to consider. The focus should be on identifying the qualities that make a great doctor and ensuring those qualities are in the applicant pool.

Before diving into this topic, to truly understand the problem with medical school admissions as it pertains to diversity, we must first ask ourselves why we want to admit students from diverse backgrounds. A standard answer is that diversity provides more opportunities for students from underrepresented backgrounds. Yes, this is true; however, it's not the primary concern and definitely not the primary reason for me writing this book. I believe the reason for admitting students from diverse backgrounds into medical school is to meet the demands of society. The purpose is not necessarily to give John or Sarah an opportunity to live out their dreams. That is just a nice byproduct of the process.

As discussed earlier, the United States is becoming more diverse, with research suggesting that a more diverse physician workforce improves the health of everyone. After hearing this, the question should be, "Why?" Certainly, it's not an intelligence issue. As a matter of fact, I believe we are truly all of one race; the human race. So, it can't be that minorities are inherently smarter than the majority race. There has to be another reason.

Here's a thought. To compete and survive in America, minorities have had to develop and hone their social skills in unique ways. When we consider the history of slavery for Black Americans, we know that opportunities for formal education were severely limited, and access to traditional avenues of advancement based solely on book smarts was denied. Instead, black individuals were forced to rely on a multitude of intangible qualities that allowed them to provide value to their communities in different ways.

Throughout generations, these intangible qualities have been prioritized and cultivated within black communities, serving as invaluable assets. Traits such as resilience, adaptability, resourcefulness, and a deep sense of community have been nurtured and passed down through generations, enabling individuals to navigate systemic barriers and create opportunities where none existed. These qualities have been essential for survival and progress, propelling individuals forward in the face of adversity. These are the same qualities that translate into excellent patient care and improved outcomes.

Sadly, despite their immense value, these qualities are often overlooked or undervalued in traditional admission decisions. Academic achievements and standardized test scores tend to take precedence, inadvertently neglecting the wealth of unique experiences and strengths that diverse candidates bring to the table. By failing to recognize and appreciate the social skills developed by minority groups, we miss out on a crucial dimension of excellence in the medical field.

Historically, medical schools have relied heavily on metrics such as grade point averages and Medical College Admission Test (MCAT) scores to evaluate applicants. These metrics have been viewed as a proxy for intelligence, but in reality, they only measure a limited aspect of an applicant's abilities. While they may be helpful in predicting academic success, they are not necessarily an indicator of clinical competence or the ability to provide compassionate care.

In today's technological age, medical knowledge is more readily available than ever before. As a result, it's essential for doctors to be resourceful and able to quickly access and apply relevant information. This means that the ability to use technology to find answers is just as important as memorization and book smarts. However, measuring this quality is not as straightforward as evaluating grades or test scores. Ultimately, we must look beyond the numbers.

One way to address this challenge is to redefine what is meant by merit in medical school admissions. Instead of focusing solely on academic performance, we also need to consider other factors that contribute to a well-rounded applicant. For example, resilience and resourcefulness are qualities that make for an exceptional doctor. When considering merit-based admissions, it is crucial to take into account the individual's experiences and the obstacles they have overcome. Students who have faced adversity, whether it be personal, financial, or academic, have often developed a unique set of skills and characteristics that are valuable in the medical field. These individuals have demonstrated a unique determination, which is an essential quality for successful physicians.

Measuring the distance traveled by an individual, in terms of their personal growth and development, can serve as a valuable criterion for merit. For example, a student who has faced financial hardship and worked multiple jobs to support their education, or a student who has had to care for a sick family member while pursuing their education, has likely developed strong time management skills, empathy, and a sense of responsibility that will translate well into their future medical practice.

When selecting medical students based on distance traveled, we must recognize that academic performance and test scores are not the only indicators of a student's potential. While GPA and MCAT scores may provide some insight into a student's ability to succeed academically, they do not necessarily reflect their potential to be an exceptional physician.

I cannot recall a single time a patient or family member asked me what my MCAT score was. I can't recall being asked what my GPA was. As a matter of fact, I can't recall a patient or family member even asking me where I went to medical school. The simple truth is they don't care. What I have been asked is, "Can you do everything possible to help my dad." I've been asked, "Will you treat them like they were your own family." That's what patients and family members care about; how far their doctor is willing to go in order to help them. They don't care about MCAT scores and GPA. Yes, I agree those are important; however, it's critical we don't overvalue the numbers and make them the end all be all.

Ultimately, by considering distance traveled as a criterion for merit, medical schools can identify and select a more diverse group of students who possess a range of valuable qualities and experiences. This approach to merit can lead to the selection of individuals who are not only academically qualified but also possess the resilience, resourcefulness, and empathy needed to succeed in the medical field and serve their communities.

Admissions Committees

Years back, I had the opportunity to serve on an admissions committee. Among the many applicants, one stood out to me, a black woman who seemed to have struggled at various stages of her academic journey. As we scrutinized her application, it became clear that if we were to judge her on numbers alone, she might not have deserved to gain acceptance. However, something about that didn't sit right with me.

As the only black individual on the committee, I felt a responsibility to go the extra mile and find the diamonds in her past. It was clear to me that she not only deserved to be in the program, but she would also be one of our best. I argued on her behalf, seemingly kicking against the goads while making a case for her candidacy. Thankfully, the case proved to be strong enough, and she was selected. As I suspected, she turned out to be among the best students in the program.

It's unfortunate that situations like this are not uncommon in healthcare and beyond. Often, individuals are overlooked because they don't fit the conventional mold or they don't have the same opportunities as others. This is where having individuals from diverse backgrounds take part in admission decision-making is crucial. When people have shared experiences, they can better appreciate the distance traveled and understand that merit is not just about numbers but also about character traits that are difficult to measure.

As I reflect on that situation, I wonder where this young lady would be if I had not been on that panel. Would she have missed out on this great opportunity that could be life-changing? Would the program have missed out on having this amazing student who undoubtedly contributed to the academic and personal development of her peers? This is why it's essential to recognize the importance of diversity in decision-making to ensure that every deserving individual has a legitimate chance to succeed.

Various studies have shown that having diversity on admissions committees can lead to a more fair and successful selection process. One study conducted by the Association of American Medical Colleges found that when admissions committees were more diverse, they were more likely to admit a diverse group of students. Specifically, they found that when at least one committee member was from a racial or ethnic minority group, the odds of admitting underrepresented minority students increased 5.3 fold.

Another study conducted by researchers at the University of Michigan found that diversity on admissions committees improves the quality of decisions made. Diverse committees were more likely to consider a broader range of criteria when evaluating applicants and were less likely to rely solely on standardized test scores. This is important because it suggests that a diverse group of decision-makers may be more likely to see the potential in students who don't fit the traditional mold.

It's important that the reader understands I am not lobbying to trade excellence for diversity. Yes, it's clear that having a diverse group of decision-makers is essential for promoting equity and social justice, but it's also crucial for ensuring that the best and most deserving candidates are selected. By having individuals from different backgrounds and perspectives on admissions committees, we can increase the likelihood that all students are given fair consideration and that the most promising candidates are admitted.

Ultimately, if we are to achieve a diverse medical workforce, we must acknowledge that our current medical admissions process is flawed and needs reform. We need to expand our criteria of merit beyond test scores and grades and consider the unique experiences and backgrounds of each applicant. Additionally, we need to diversify admissions committees to ensure that they reflect the diversity of our society and can make more informed and unbiased decisions. Most importantly, we need to focus on the needs of our patients and train healthcare professionals who can provide culturally competent care to diverse populations. Until we can accomplish these tasks, we risk perpetuating health disparities and leaving talented individuals out of the medical profession.

Chapter 7

DIVERSIFYING ACADEMIC MEDICINE

"A PUPIL IS NOT above his teacher, but everyone, after he has been fully trained, will be like his teacher." – Luke 6:40

When you think about the Los Angeles Lakers, which superstar comes to mind? Magic? Kareem? Shaq? West? For me, it's Kobe Bryant, one of the greatest basketball players to walk the earth. This megastar didn't get there on his own. Among the many individuals he learned from, Michael Jordan stands out as one of the most influential. From a young age, Kobe watched Jordan's moves and studied them as meticulously as he could. Kobe even went to the extent of hiring Jordan's same trainer. Eventually, Jordan became one of Kobe's more revered mentors, and the relationship morphed into big brother – little brother. The result of this teacher-student relationship was a near-identical style of play, twin-like mindsets, and an awful lot of championship rings.

Medicine is no different. As doctors, we, too, must be educated at the feet of individuals more established and advanced than we are. Nobody learns to cut open a body and transplant a heart without a bit of guidance along the way. But how does diversity play a role in this guidance? This is a question worth asking and answering. Thus far in this book, we've discussed the lack of diversity in the medical field and its implications; however, we're yet to narrow the focus to academic medicine specifically. Let's take a moment to consider this.

When I walk the hallways of my hospital, I'm fully aware that I'm a unicorn. By that, I mean I'm a rare sighting.   There aren't very many black doctors, let alone black male doctors, on faculty. According to the Association of American Medical Colleges 2022 Data Report, while underrepresented minority groups make up approximately 32% of the U.S. population, they account for only around 12% of full-time medical school faculty and 12% of permanent medical school deans. Narrowing the focus, Black/African American individuals comprise roughly 13% of the U.S. population but constitute just 4% of full-time medical school faculty and only 2% of medical school deans. Hispanic/Latino individuals face a similar underrepresentation, with around 18% of the population but only 6% of full-time medical school faculty and 4% of medical school deans.

The consequences of subpar diversity in academic medicine are far-reaching. In medical school, having teachers from minority and diverse backgrounds is crucial. They bring unique perspectives, cultural insights, and personal experiences that can educate future healthcare professionals about the social determinants of health and the factors that contribute to healthcare disparities.

Consider Dr. Johnson, an African American physician and medical school faculty member. Dr. Johnson was raised to carry a certain level of pride for her black heritage. Her parents educated her on their rich family history and cultural practices, much of which directly or indirectly impact health. Dr. Johnson, being raised in this manner and in a community with others holding shared practices, is well equipped to educate students on the nuances pertaining to caring for populations similar to her own. By sharing her personal experiences and insights, she can help students better understand the challenges faced by some minority populations, thereby better preparing them with the knowledge needed to address health disparities effectively.

The importance of diversity in academic medicine extends beyond medical education. Academic physicians also serve as role models and mentors for trainees, shaping their professional development and influencing their career paths. Take a moment to think back to your childhood. There are probably a few teachers or coaches that you have fond memories of. Individuals that you believed played a critical role in you getting to where you are today. These are people you admired and could see your future self in. People you wanted to emulate to some extent. Even if you didn't want to do exactly what they did for a living, something about them was inspirational and helped shape you to become the person you are.

In my case, one such example was my soccer coach, who left a lasting impact on me. His name was Larry Hope. To this day, I tell my children about Coach Hope. When I think about my childhood, beyond family, there are few people I recall going out of their way to help me in a manner I would consider significant. Coach Hope was one of them. My parents often worked too late to get me to soccer practice on time. Coach Hope would pick me up on a regular basis just to ensure I could have the experience like the other kids. During the games, I was the annoying kid that never wanted to sit out. I'd walk up and down the sidelines like his shadow, constantly asking if I could go back in the game. I don't recall a single time Coach Hope got upset with me. He was always kind and patient and would promise to get me in the game when able. Now that I think about it, Coach Hope was the only black male coach I recall having.

As I'm writing this, I'm literally on a flight to my medical school alma mater, where they will be hosting me for one of my Black Men In White Coats youth summits. Although I'm incredibly excited to see the kids and positively impact their lives, I'm just as excited to see my mentor, Dr. Ellis Ingram. Dr. Ingram was one of four black male faculty members I remember during the eight years I spent in Missouri for undergrad and medical school. Like Coach Hope, Dr. Ingram went out of his way to ensure I was taken care of. And not just me; he did this for as many students as would come to him, regardless of their race. It turns out, however, that many of the students who took advantage of this were minorities. For eight years, Dr. Ingram looked out for me, and he continues to do so to this day.

When trainees see doctors who share similar backgrounds and experiences in positions of leadership, authority, and expertise, they are more likely to envision themselves in those roles. Seeing Dr. Ingram helped me vicariously explore academic medicine as a career. It also led me to focus my efforts on uplifting the next generation of physician leaders. In all my years in Missouri, I recall just one or two lectures he gave me, yet he was my most influential professor. In so many ways, he showed me the right path. Much of this was passive, and he unknowingly guided me to places I otherwise may not have considered had it not been for me watching the way in which he carried himself. As a black man, I viewed him to be like me; he was relatable. I felt more connected with him than with other faculty, and his successes gave me a certain level of confidence that I could go off and do great things in the field of medicine.

Academic medicine needs more doctors like Ellis Ingram. Individuals from diverse backgrounds who are not only teaching from a unique perspective but also walking as role models. Appreciating the importance of such individuals is only the starting point. The real question then becomes, what are the barriers to increasing the numbers and getting greater diversity in academic medicine?

Money Talks

Thinking back to medical school and residency, I recall so many of my friends who were interested in pursuing careers in academic medicine. Their mission was to teach the next generation of clinician leaders and help shape the healthcare landscape. However, when it came time to make the decision between private practice and academic medicine, their dreams of impacting academic medicine vanished as they chose private careers. Even now, as I watch residents and fellows progress through their training, I see the same pattern.

There are many divides between the worlds of academic medicine and private practice. Among the most obvious are financial incentives. Young doctors are often faced with the choice between pursuing a career in academic medicine, where they can make a difference in research, mentorship, and education, or private practice, where they can earn significantly more money. That's not to say you can't make money in academic medicine or have an educational impact in private practice, but for the most part, those are the reasons doctors choose one of these two career paths. In the end, it's the immense compensation disparity that has led many doctors to choose private practice over academic medicine, and this is a significant reason why we continue to struggle to increase diversity in academic medicine.

For many doctors, the decision to go into private practice is a simple one. After many grueling years of medical school, residency, and fellowship, they understandably want to be compensated for their hard work. The prospect of earning a mid to high six-figure salary is enticing, especially for those who have accrued significant student debt. Who can blame any of these doctors for choosing a more lucrative career path, as they have bills to pay and families to support? Although I'm in academic medicine, I'd be lying if I said I haven't thought about private practice on a few occasions.

Let's examine this hypothetical situation of two young doctors, one pursuing academic medicine and the other private practice. Dr. A has completed a three-year internal medicine residency and is considering an academic position as a hospitalist. The starting salary for this position is $150,000 per year. Dr. B, on the other hand, has decided to join a private practice group in the same city. As a primary care physician, Dr. B can expect to earn a starting salary of $250,000 per year. In a few years, Dr. B will have the opportunity to become a partner in the group and, in doing so, nearly triple his salary. The financial difference between the two positions is significant, and it's not hard to see why Dr. B might be more inclined to choose private practice.

This financial divide may be even more important for minority doctors. In some cases, these doctors come from lower-income families and are burdened with greater student debt. For them, the incentives of private practice are even more compelling.

Imagine growing up in poverty in the projects of the south side of Chicago. Your parents work relentlessly to put you in a position for academic success so you have a chance to attend junior college. After completing two years of junior college, you transition to a four-year institution which is much more expensive.

Your parents can't afford the tuition, so you take out loans. A couple years pass, and although you tried your best, you struggle to get a decent score on the MCAT and therefore opt to take a few gap years. To boost your candidacy for medical school, you enroll in a post-baccalaureate program that costs almost as much as your undergraduate tuition. After your prolonged journey, you finally gain admission to medical school, where you again must take out an excessive amount of student loans. Through it all, although your parents possess an unconditional love for you, they can't support you financially. As a matter of fact, you've been using your loans to help support them.

Fast forward a few years, and you're now completing your neurosurgery residency, which took an additional seven years post-medical school. Two job options are presented to you. The first is for an academic medicine position in which you are being offered a salary of $400,000. You're excited and think that's great money since your total school loan debt is just a little more than that at $500,000. Then, the local private practice group approaches you with a salary offer of $750,000. Which one are you choosing? I get it; many of you would say it depends on the specific job roles and your goals. I'd agree with that; however, this example illustrates why for many docs, particularly those from specific upbringings, the private option could be the right choice.

Some people would argue that academic medicine is a noble career, and money should not be the goal. While this may be true, the reality is that money matters. Doctors have worked hard over the years, and when they are done with their training, they expect to be compensated accordingly. The problem is that the financial incentives in academic medicine are not as attractive as those in private practice. This is a complex problem to solve, as the funding for academic medicine is often tied to grants and government funding, which are not always reliable.

In my case, the call to academia won, although it took some work to get me there. In 2016, I completed my fellowship training in Pulmonary & Critical Care Medicine. I had a growing family and a significant amount of debt hanging over my head. As both my wife and I were doctors, the debt problem was a double whammy, and finding jobs that paid well was crucial to our financial stability. I was being recruited to a relatively new hospital in which I was being given the opportunity to build their ICU program while earning more money than I had ever imagined being offered for practicing medicine. To say the least, this seemed like a no-brainer decision for us; I had to take the job.

Just before I signed the contract, the chairman of our department, whom I greatly admired for his intellect and leadership, summoned me to his office to discuss my future. Subsequently,

I met with my division chief and one of my mentors who served in an Assistant Dean role. As we talked, they opened my eyes to the idea that I could have a significant impact in the field of academic medicine. Their insight and recommendations made me consider pursuing this path instead of the private gig. By describing unique attributes they had identified in me over the years, they were able to demonstrate my specific role in shaping the future of medicine. They recognized that I would be an asset not only to the department but to healthcare as a whole, and my vehicle for doing that could be academic medicine.

While their recognition of these things was meaningful, what's most important is they used them as strategies to recruit me and increase diversity in academic medicine. Despite the financial implications, they helped me to realize that academia was where I could make a significant impact and find true fulfillment in my work. Years later, I'm so grateful for those meetings, as they led me to a career that has been more rewarding than I imagined.

Considering my journey, I'm convinced that one thing we must become better at in academic medicine is recruiting excellence from diverse backgrounds. If we hope to increase diversity in healthcare and establish a culturally proficient system, we need teachers that will be mindful of the issues at hand and take the lead to rectify them. Ultimately, because money talks, recruiting such talent will likely require higher compensation in academic medicine across the board, regardless of one's race. It's a real expense, but the cost of not getting this right could be a lot more.

Taxation Without Representation

"It's too much! I'm about to quit!"

These are the words I vented to the president of a Historically Black College and University (HBCU) some years back. I was referring to the amount of work that was put on me as a young faculty member. In reality, most of it was not required by my institution; however, they had asked me to serve in specific capacities, and as one of the few black doctors, I felt obligated to represent others who looked like me. That being the case, I accepted many of the roles.

However, as burnout transformed from a theory to reality in my life, I reached the point where I was ready to quit. Not quit my job but the various roles and responsibilities I had been entrusted with. While I enjoyed the roles, I was not sure how they would impact my professional development and, more importantly, my home life as my children were growing older. For me, being present in their lives was of utmost importance, and I was approaching a fork in the road. I was convinced my overall workload, clinical and nonclinical combined, was far greater than what my friends in private practice were experiencing.

This was my fork in the road. Do I stay in academic medicine or transition to private practice?

Fortunately, this president gave me superb guidance. She encouraged me to stay in the fight and reminded me that while it's a true responsibility, it's also an honored opportunity to represent others in the capacities I was afforded. She provided many great pieces of advice that I have since employed for my productivity and sanity. Perhaps the most important thing I learned from her was how to prioritize. She emphasized the importance of knowing where I should focus my efforts and learning how to say 'no' to everything else that would drain my time with minimal yield.

As I write this, 2 Chronicles 15:7 comes to mind. "But as for you, be strong and do not give up, for your work will be rewarded."

Years removed from that conversation, I have been rewarded for staying in the fight and continuing in my various roles. Within my institution, my efforts have been acknowledged with awards, leadership opportunities, and promotion in academic rank. At the same time, learning to prioritize and say 'no' has allowed me to be present at home with my wife and children. My purpose in sharing this story is to highlight the importance of counseling, advising, and mentorship for young faculty members, and more specifically, minority junior faculty. Had I not received astute direction from a more accomplished academic clinician, I may not be where I am today.

This story of increased burdens is not unique to me. In academia, minority doctors often find themselves disproportionately burdened with responsibilities related to diversity and inclusion. These additional tasks range from serving on diversity committees to participating in recruitment efforts, mentoring minority students, and addressing issues related to healthcare disparities. Although these initiatives are crucial for creating inclusive environments and addressing systemic injustices, they come with significant time and energy investments. Unfortunately, these efforts are often unpaid or inadequately compensated, creating an additional strain on minority doctors' professional and personal lives.

The lack of diversity in leadership positions at academic medical centers further exacerbates this issue. When the individuals shaping institutional policies and decision-making lack diverse perspectives, it falls upon minority faculty to bear the responsibility of advocating for change and representing the interests of underrepresented communities. This dynamic places an unfair burden on minority doctors, as we are tasked with navigating the challenges of our own career progression while simultaneously addressing issues of diversity and inclusion.

Let's take a moment to revisit history. In the 18th century, American colonies were under British rule, and the British government imposed various taxes on the colonists without granting them a say in the decisions made in the British Parliament. This meant that the colonists had no voice in the laws and policies that directly impacted their lives, particularly when it came to taxation. Naturally, this sparked deep resentment and frustration among the colonists, leading to the popular slogan "no taxation without representation." This phrase captured the belief that individuals should have the right to be heard and to participate in shaping the laws that govern them, especially in matters of taxation. It became a rallying cry during the American Revolution, and it laid the groundwork for the principles of democracy and self-determination that formed the basis of the birth of the United States of America.

The disproportionate burden of diversity work placed on minorities has been aptly termed the "minority tax." Just as the colonist faced taxation without representation, minority doctors find themselves shouldering an extra workload (i.e., the tax), often without commensurate support, compensation, or recognition. The minority tax creates a challenging environment in academic medicine where involved doctors and staff feel as though their voices and concerns are undervalued or overlooked. It is a barrier that hampers their ability to focus on career advancement and professional growth, as they are often consumed, and in some cases sidetracked, by the demands of diversity work.

The implications of this minority tax are far-reaching. It can create a situation where institutions inadvertently perpetuate the cycle of unequal representation and limited progress. The taxing nature of this burden dissuades many young minority doctors from pursuing academic medicine, as they perceive private practice as a more conducive environment for career advancement and personal fulfillment. The minority tax can also slow the progression of junior faculty to senior levels of leadership, where it may be easier for them to promote their efforts and enact change.

To rectify this issue, it is crucial for academic medical centers to address the root causes of the minority tax. Institutions should prioritize the creation of diverse leadership teams, ensuring that decision-making bodies reflect the populations they serve. By distributing the responsibility of diversity work more equitably across the medical community, institutions can foster a collaborative and inclusive environment that better fosters career progression for all doctors, regardless of their background.

Furthermore, institutions should provide appropriate compensation and support for the extra workload associated with diversity work. By compensation, I mean both monetary and merit acknowledgment toward academic promotion. Recognizing the value and impact of these efforts, both in terms of promoting equity and enhancing the learning environment, is vital. In valuing the contributions of minority doctors and acknowledging the challenges they face, institutions can create an environment where diversity and inclusion are shared responsibilities rather than shouldered by a few.

Until we move beyond "taxation without representation," it seems likely that diversity in academic medicine will remain relatively stagnant. This, in turn, will limit our ability to address healthcare disparities and optimize our medical system for everyone.

Chapter 8

REDUCING
ATTRITION

I T PAINS MY HEART each time I see a minority colleague
leave academic medicine. While I understand their reasoning and want the best for them, I often find myself working to
convince them to stay. Undoubtedly, there's a selfish motive behind my efforts, as I would like to avoid the feeling of isolation.
But in the end, my efforts tend to fall short. Once their minds
are made up, there's little that can be done.

The reality we face is that URM faculty members are leaving academic medicine at a higher rate compared to their
non-URM counterparts. This departure is happening on top of
existing discrepancies in faculty representation, which are also
reflected in healthcare outcomes. These numbers, though significant, go beyond mere statistics. Each departing faculty member takes with them a valuable set of experiences and perspectives that could have enriched the learning environment and
patient care for students, colleagues, staff, and patients alike.

Appreciating this disparity in attrition, the next question would be, why are minorities leaving academia at higher rates. It does little good to know that the problem exists unless you have a mechanism to solve it. To develop that mechanism, understanding the 'why' is essential. In this case, there is a multitude of reasons, perhaps too many to cover. At the end of the day, however, I believe it comes down to two primary issues.

Inadequate Support

Let's start with a lack of support towards goals. Recently, I had a meeting with a doctor who served as an Associate Dean of Diversity at her medical school. For the sake of anonymity, let's call her Dr. Jones. Dr. Jones was the real deal and had worked her way up the ladder to earn this position. She was so fired up about healthcare disparities, medical education, and being a part of the revolution that would take us beyond the status quo. If anyone seemed ready to take on the challenge, it was her. Well, that's what I thought until she quit her job and left academia altogether.

Perplexed by her decision, I probed and was finally able to get to the source. Dr. Jones, in a sense, felt that she was there for show, a token of sorts. She had so many great ideas and was eager to implement them. Avant-garde, she believed she could revolutionize diversity's impact on healthcare, but the support simply was not there. Yes, it's great to be put in a position of power, but is it really power if it's void of resources? In the end, Dr. Jones concluded that the institution did not honestly care about diversity. How could they? After all, as she saw it, they had set her up for failure.

Embarking on a career dedicated to fostering diversity within academic medicine is no easy task. The landscape of promotions and career progression in this field is deeply intertwined with scholarly work, particularly research grants and publications. However, for many underrepresented minority faculty members who aspire to make a meaningful impact on diversity, there is a prevailing sense of urgency—an "act now" mentality.

URM faculty members often prioritize the implementation of programs and initiatives that yield short-term results, aiming to address health disparities and the lack of diversity in medicine. However, the execution of such programs relies heavily on securing adequate resources, which can prove challenging to obtain within the confines of academia. Dr. Jones's experience serves as a perfect illustration of this predicament.

Despite being granted a leadership position, Dr. Jones found herself facing resistance when it came to securing the necessary resources to turn her ideas into reality. In many ways, she had an uphill climb. The limited support received hampered her chances of success in her role and severely constrained her opportunities for career advancement. Frustrated by this lack of support and recognizing the dwindling prospects for success, she made the difficult decision to escape the mounting stress and depart from academia.

Dr. Jones's story reflects the immense challenges faced by URM faculty members who endeavor to make a lasting impact on diversity within academic medicine. The scarcity of resources, both financial and structural, poses a significant hurdle to their ability to effect meaningful change. The mismatch between the urgency of their aspirations and the slow-moving nature of academia creates a sense of frustration and disillusionment, leading many talented individuals to seek alternative paths outside of their academic institutions.

While the pursuit of immediate impact and tangible change is commendable, it is essential to address the underlying issues that perpetuate this cycle of frustration and attrition among URM faculty members. Academic institutions must recognize the need for a paradigm shift in evaluating success and career advancement within the realm of diversity. This shift involves redefining the criteria for promotion and acknowledging the value of community engagement, program implementation, and the creation of inclusive environments as vital contributions to healthcare.

Moreover, it is incumbent upon academic institutions to allocate adequate resources and funding to support initiatives ultimately aimed at advancing diversity and reducing healthcare disparities. By providing URM faculty members with the necessary tools and support systems, institutions can empower them to execute their vision and effect real change via academic medicine. This leads to job satisfaction, and job satisfaction leads to retention.

Career Progression

Related to inadequate support, a second notable reason URM faculty are leaving academic medicine is the lack of career progression. Multiple studies highlight the significant gaps in promotion rates between URM and non-URM faculty. For instance, a study published in the Journal of General Internal Medicine found that URM faculty were 22% less likely to be promoted to the rank of associate professor compared to their non-URM counterparts. Another study published in JAMA Internal Medicine revealed that URM faculty had a 27% lower likelihood of achieving promotion to the rank of full professor compared to non-URM faculty. These statistics underscore the pronounced disparities in career advancement faced by URM faculty members. Understanding the underlying barriers that impede promotions is crucial in addressing the inequities within academic medicine.

Inadequate Mentorship

Effective mentorship is vital for career development and success in academic medicine. It provides invaluable support, guidance, and insights into navigating the intricate pathways of the academic landscape. However, URM faculty often find themselves facing significant barriers in accessing mentors who genuinely understand their unique experiences and can offer tailored guidance.

Mentors play a crucial role in fostering professional development, expanding research opportunities, and connecting individuals to influential networks. They provide guidance on securing research grants, publishing papers, and navigating the complex landscape of promotions. The lack of diversity among mentors who have successfully advanced through the ranks represents a critical gap in the support system for URM faculty. These mentors are invaluable for providing insight into the unwritten rules, expectations, and strategies required for career progression. They have firsthand experience with the challenges and barriers URM individuals uniquely encounter, and without them, it becomes challenging to receive the guidance necessary for promotion. As a result, inequities in promotion perpetuate.

Addressing the challenge of inadequate mentorship and guidance requires proactive efforts. Implementing mentorship programs specifically designed to support URM faculty and recruiting diverse mentors can help bridge the gap. These programs should focus on providing URM faculty with the necessary guidance, support, and opportunities for networking and professional growth. Additionally, mentorship training programs for faculty members can help cultivate the skills needed to effectively mentor URM individuals, fostering a culture of inclusive mentorship within academic medicine.

Limited Networks

"Show me your five closest friends, and I'll show you your future." – Jim Rohn

Next, let's consider the limited networking opportunities URM faculty may have and how this impacts promotion. Networking is a cornerstone of academic promotions, as it enables individuals to establish critical connections, gain visibility, and secure support from influential colleagues. However, URM faculty often encounter limited networking opportunities, which hinders their ability to expand their professional circles and cultivate supportive relationships.

A significant contributor factor to the limited networking opportunities faced by URM faculty is the thought-provoking phenomenon explored in Dr. Beverly Daniel Tatum's book, "Why Do All the Black Kids Sit Together at Lunch?" This book delves into the dynamics of racial identity development and the impact of socialization patterns among diverse individuals. Dr. Tatum, a highly respected psychologist and former president of Spelman College, presents a compelling analysis of the challenges faced by URM individuals in predominantly white institutions.

The book delves into the complexities of racial identity formation and the tendency for URM individuals to seek solace and camaraderie within their own racial or ethnic groups. This phenomenon, commonly observed in schools, workplaces, and various social settings, can be attributed to a variety of factors, including shared experiences, cultural affinity, and the need for support in environments where URM individuals may feel marginalized or underrepresented.

While these gatherings and spaces can provide a sense of community and support, they also present a unique challenge for URM faculty who aspire to expand their networks beyond their own racial boundaries. Breaking away from the comfort and familiarity of socializing within one's racial or ethnic group requires intentional effort and the development of cross-cultural communication skills.

Dr. Tatum's work prompts us to reflect on the broader implications of this phenomenon within the context of academic medicine. URM faculty members, who often find themselves in environments with limited racial diversity, face the additional challenge of navigating networking spaces that are predominantly occupied by colleagues from different racial backgrounds. This dynamic creates a need for URM faculty to bridge cultural gaps, overcome potential biases, and build connections across racial boundaries to enhance their professional growth and advancement opportunities.

While it is crucial to acknowledge the significance of affinity spaces for URM individuals and the empowerment they can provide, it is equally important to recognize the potential limitations they may impose on networking opportunities. Encouraging dialogue and fostering inclusive environments that promote cross-cultural connections can help address this challenge.

The ability to code-switch is of utmost importance for URM faculty members seeking to build their networks within academic medicine. Code-switching refers to the skill of adapting communication styles and behaviors to effectively navigate diverse social settings. URM faculty members often find themselves in institutions where the prevailing communication norms may differ from their own cultural backgrounds. This skill allows them to bridge these cultural gaps, effectively engage with colleagues from diverse backgrounds, and establish connections necessary for career advancement.

For some individuals, code-switching comes with an internal conflict. They fear that they are compromising their authenticity or "selling out." It is essential to recognize that code-switching is not a betrayal of one's true self. On the contrary, it is an admirable skill that showcases adaptability and the ability to navigate different cultural and professional contexts. Code-switching allows URM faculty members to bring their authentic selves to various settings while effectively communicating and building meaningful connections with colleagues from different backgrounds.

By mastering the art of code-switching, URM faculty members can better navigate networking opportunities, engage in collaborations, and garner support from influential individuals within academic medicine. It is a strategic and necessary tool to break through potential barriers and access the resources and opportunities that can propel their careers forward.

Bias and Stereotypes

In addition to the challenges already mentioned, we must address the persistence of implicit biases and stereotypes within academic medicine that negatively impact the promotion process for URM faculty. Despite efforts to foster diversity and inclusivity, bias continues to infiltrate the evaluation and decision-making processes, influencing promotion outcomes.

Implicit biases are unconscious associations and attitudes that individuals hold, which can affect their perceptions and judgments. These biases, often ingrained through societal norms and stereotypes, can shape how URM faculty members are evaluated and hinder their professional achievements. For example, a stereotype that URM individuals may not possess the same level of competence or expertise as their non-URM counterparts can taint the evaluation process, leading to lower expectations and biased assessments.

I'm reminded of an instance that happened to me on one specific clinical rotation. At the time, I was a senior trainee responsible for supervising a junior resident. One morning, during our rounds, our attending physician began showering the resident with profuse praises and exclaimed their astonishment at the resident's ability to handle complex cases and deliver exceptional care. From the outside, it appeared to be a well-deserved compliment, but there was more to the story than met the eye. The reality was some of the credit should have been attributed to the work I was quietly performing. Yet, I chose not to disclose that I was the one laboring behind the scenes, because I did not want to dim the resident's shine.

Late nights, I would meticulously review the resident's tasks, ensuring accuracy and rectifying any errors. I didn't think much of this as it was my responsibility. From adjusting antibiotics to ordering the appropriate lab tests, I diligently worked to maintain the highest standard of care for our patients. Despite this, I never received comparable feedback or recognition. Nonetheless, I wasn't bothered because acknowledgment was never my motive; rather, my focus was to deliver exceptional care to my patients.

It wasn't until one particular incident that the situation truly began to bother me. I had a meeting with an individual in leadership at our institution. This individual shared with me that my supervising doctor had contacted them, reporting they were concerned with the way I handled a specific patient situation. The individual who was sharing this information with me was quite confused as they had recruited me to the institution and knew me to be a hard worker with strong clinical acumen. They simply could not comprehend how that feedback could be accurate, and neither could I.

After taking a deeper dive into the case, it became evident what the issue was. My supervising doctor was gone for a few days, and their colleague took charge of the service. With that came a slightly divergent plan of care, which I followed as instructed. It wasn't that I was going against my attending doctor's plan of care; what truly happened was their colleague had a different plan which I carried out. This situation has weighed heavily on my mind, and this is the first time I have since discussed it. It left me to question how the supervising doctor arrived at the conclusion, which they did.

I've debated in my mind for years if I'm being too sensitive about this topic. I try to convince myself it's not a big deal and that, in the grand scheme of things, that was a little issue. But was it? I'm bothered by the fact that with all the work I did, and the credit given to someone else, an attempt to inappropriately throw me under the bus was made. Throughout my medical training, I performed rather well and typically received exceptional evaluations.

Interestingly enough, this individual still gave me a good evaluation which further bothered me. Why would you report something to my leadership but never tell me? If you were concerned about my management decisions, why not ask me? Why would you provide positive written feedback rather than share with me your concerns so I could improve? This person led me to believe they thought I did a good job, but behind the scenes, they tried to pull me down.

This disheartening experience serves as a stark reminder of how biases and preconceived notions can hinder the career advancement of URM doctors in academic medicine. I can't prove that these were factors in my case; however, I highly suspect so. Despite my dedicated efforts and role in ensuring superb patient care, I witnessed what appeared to be my attending physician's implicit bias play out before my eyes. The resident, who I supervised and supported, received tremendous praise and admiration, while my contributions went unnoticed and unacknowledged. Day in and day out, I sat there and watched my attending champion this resident and set them on a pedestal. Nothing of the like was ever directed to me, even though I carried the load for the team. Sure, it's possible my supervising physician simply didn't notice, but my question would be, how not?

This situation highlights the insidious impact of biases on the trajectory of URM doctors' careers. When these biases are at play, deserving individuals may be overlooked and undervalued, and their accomplishments overshadowed or attributed to others. Such disparities in recognition and advancement can have profound consequences on the professional development and overall well-being of URM doctors. I'm a prime example of that. Years later, this event still bothers me.

Such incidents as mine occur on a daily basis. The lack of acknowledgment not only robs URM faculty of the credit they deserve but also perpetuates systemic inequities within academic medicine. When biases influence promotion decisions, it undermines the principles of fairness, meritocracy, and equal opportunities. Just imagine if I were up for a promotion at that time when my attending presented off-record to essentially discredit my abilities? On paper, they supported me, but untraced, they told a different story.

Moreover, the repercussions of biased career advancement extend beyond the individual. The attrition rates among URM doctors in academic medicine are already concerning, and experiences like mine only exacerbate this issue. The sense of being undervalued and unseen can contribute to burnout and a desire to leave academic medicine altogether, worsening the underrepresentation of URM faculty.

Stereotypes also play a role in perpetuating systemic inequities. Stereotypes such as the "model minority" myth, which suggests that certain racial and ethnic groups are naturally high achievers, can create unrealistic expectations and put additional pressure on URM faculty to constantly prove themselves. On the other hand, stereotypes that associate URM individuals with negative attributes or assume that they are less competent can undermine their professional achievements and hinder their advancement opportunities.

The impact of biases and stereotypes extends beyond subjective evaluations. Promotion decisions that do not solely rely on merit and scholarly accomplishments can perpetuate systemic inequities and create barriers for URM faculty members. The reliance on subjective assessments, influenced by implicit biases, may lead to inconsistencies and unfair treatment in promotion decisions. URM faculty members may find themselves overlooked or undervalued, despite their significant contributions to research, teaching, and patient care.

Addressing this requires a multifaceted approach. Academic institutions must implement strategies to raise awareness about implicit biases and foster a culture of inclusivity and fairness. Providing unconscious bias training to faculty members involved in promotion decisions can help mitigate the impact of biases on evaluations. Creating clear and objective evaluation criteria based on measurable outcomes may also reduce the influence of subjective assessments.

Furthermore, establishing diverse promotion and tenure committees can also contribute to fair and unbiased evaluations. Ensuring that committee members come from diverse backgrounds and possess cultural competency can challenge biases and promote a more equitable promotion process. Also, it is crucial for programs to create avenues for feedback and transparency in promotion decisions, allowing faculty members to address any concerns or biases that may have influenced their evaluations.

Ultimately, if we want to move towards a more excellent healthcare system, the issue of URM advancement in academic medicine must be appropriately addressed. The consequences of inequitable promotions within academic medicine are far-reaching and detrimental to URM faculty members, the institutions themselves, and society at large. Until we address this issue, we'll continue to see an exodus of URM faculty from academia and likely worsening healthcare disparities. By recognizing and challenging the various issues mentioned in this chapter, institutions can foster a culture that values and supports the professional growth and advancement of all faculty, including the URM clinician.

Chapter 9

A LEGACY OF UNITY

"**B**E DEVOTED TO ONE another in love. Honor one another above yourselves." – Romans 12:10

On May 25, 2020, a horrific incident unfolded in Minneapolis, Minnesota, that shook the world and ignited a global movement for justice and racial equality. George Floyd, a 46-year-old Black man, encountered a tragic fate at the hands of four police officers. The sequence of events that unfolded during his arrest is a chilling testament to the injustices that persist in our society.

It began with a routine police encounter, as George Floyd was approached by officers responding to a call about an alleged counterfeit $20 bill. Within moments, the situation escalated, and George Floyd found himself pinned to the ground, his face pressed against the unforgiving pavement. Officer Derek Chauvin, with an unwavering and callous disregard for human life, knelt on George Floyd's neck for an agonizingly long eight minutes and 46 seconds.

As George Floyd pleaded for his life, gasping for breath and uttering the haunting words "I can't breathe," his cries were met with indifference from the officers involved. Bystanders who witnessed the unfolding tragedy pleaded with the officers to show mercy, to release their grip, to recognize the imminent danger to George Floyd's life. Their pleas, filled with desperation and anguish, fell on deaf ears.

George Floyd's last moments on this earth were marked by sheer terror, pain, and a cruel disregard for his humanity. The weight of the officer's knee on his neck, coupled with the indifference of those sworn to protect and serve, snuffed out a life full of dreams, aspirations, and the potential for change.

The brutal murder of George Floyd transcended boundaries, capturing the attention of the world through a gut-wrenching video that circulated on social media. The footage served as a stark and undeniable testament to the reality faced by black individuals who too often find themselves at the receiving end of systemic racism.

In the aftermath of George Floyd's murder, communities were shaken to their core, and a powerful movement demanding justice and an end to racial inequality swept through the nation. I distinctly remember receiving an influx of messages from friends and colleagues expressing genuine concern for my well-being and inquiring about how I was affected by the recent events. It wasn't just me; people across the United States who shared similar skin tones received such check-ins. And with these check-ins, the questions that kept arising were, "How can I contribute to the cause? How can I help to make things better for minorities and for America?"

Initially, I was bothered by these questions for a variety of reasons. As a natural skeptic, it was hard for me to believe so many of these people who were reaching out genuinely cared. Past experiences made me question the authenticity of intentions. I recall a particular acquaintance with whom I had a phone conversation that resulted in a disagreement about diversity efforts. Afterward, I couldn't help but feel he had only called because it was the expected thing to do, allowing him to join the bandwagon and claim he had reached out to a black friend to offer his condolences. It seemed as if checking in on me had little connection to the pain George Floyd's friends and family were enduring.

Another reason for my initial annoyance stemmed from the burden often placed on minorities. When asked how they could help, I wondered why these individuals couldn't generate their own solutions instead of relying solely on me. We had all witnessed the same tragedy, and as I grappled with its implications for my black sons and daughter, I felt overwhelmed by the expectation to provide solutions for others to get involved. It would have been more meaningful if they had taken a moment to reflect and offer their own suggestions as potential solutions.

However, with some distance from the incident, I now recognize that I may not have been fair to those who reached out. As a matter of fact, that's the entire purpose of this book. To demonstrate the power of diversity and how, with it comes new perspectives. These individuals reached out to me for my different perspective. They wanted to leverage my "diversity" to find a solution. How could I be mad at that? While I still believe some individuals did so out of obligation or as a mere checkbox exercise, I better understand how George Floyd's death created an opportunity for meaningful conversations. It was a time when people were more willing to listen to the voices of a hurting community. Initially, my responses were fueled by anger and frustration, but upon reflection, I am grateful for those who reached out and value their willingness to engage in dialogue.

Among the most profound moments I was involved with was a gathering at a local hospital. After a solemn period of silence, I was asked to step forward and share a few words. As someone very accustomed to public speaking, addressing large crowds doesn't intimidate me. However, on that day, as I stood before a sea of white coats assembled to pay respect to George Floyd and his family, I was deeply moved. I remember a slight tremor, not from fear but from a deep sense of awe. In that moment, I wholeheartedly believed that every individual present genuinely cared about what had transpired. I believed their hearts mourned with a hurting community. I believed they cared about black people. And with that, I believed they cared about me. They truly wanted to help.

I've had the fantastic privilege of dedicating my career to advancing diversity in the field of medicine, and it has been a profound honor to contribute to the betterment of our nation's health. As I reflect on my journey, I contemplate the legacy I hope to leave. Do I want to be remembered for successfully increasing the representation of black men in medicine? Or for creating widespread mentoring opportunities that empower aspiring healthcare professionals across the nation? Perhaps my genuine aspiration lies in empowering leaders to effectively impact change within their own communities. While all these accomplishments would be deeply fulfilling, there is one career goal that resonates with me on a higher level: bridging the divide between supporters and opponents of diversity efforts.

I firmly believe that beneath our perceived differences, we share more in common than we realize. Often, it is the narratives we hold and the stories we tell ourselves that shape our perceptions of the other side. If I can play a role in dismantling those barriers and fostering a sense of unity and understanding, the fight would have been worth it.

Bridging this divide requires us to challenge our own assumptions and engage in meaningful dialogue with those who hold differing views. It means acknowledging the fears, concerns, and misunderstandings that underlie resistance to diversity initiatives. By approaching these conversations with empathy and a genuine desire to listen, we can create opportunities for connection and growth. Ultimately, we don't have to agree on everything, but we can do our best to love one another.

My desire is to create a legacy of unity where diversity is celebrated as a collective strength rather than a source of division. By building bridges of understanding and finding common ground, we can create a future where diversity and inclusivity are embraced as essential pillars of a thriving healthcare system.

Anyone who truly knows me is aware of the ongoing battle I face with my own pride. It is a constant struggle for me to ask for help and to overcome the misconception that doing so is a sign of weakness. Vulnerability has never come easy to me, but I am actively working on personal growth and am determined to lay down my pride for the greater good. In the pursuit of diversifying the medical field and improving healthcare, I have come to realize that we cannot achieve meaningful progress in silos; we must work together. This means asking for help.

I sincerely appreciate and acknowledge those individuals who have reached out to offer their support and assistance. Their willingness to actively engage and contribute to this important work is commendable. Particularly for my non-URM friends, I understand the delicate balance you may perceive, wanting to be involved without stepping on anyone's toes. It is through this book that I want to express my heartfelt gratitude to all of you, regardless of race, who have extended your hands to help advance healthcare.

In moments of reflection, I find solace and inspiration in Revelation 7:9. It serves as a powerful reminder that in the grand scheme of things, we are all connected. The verse reads, "After this, I looked, and there before me was a great multitude that no one could count, from every nation, tribe, people, and language, standing before the throne and before the Lamb."

This verse encapsulates the vision of unity and inclusion that should guide our actions in diversifying the medical field and improving healthcare for all. It reminds us that the pursuit of equity and accessibility in healthcare transcends boundaries of race, ethnicity, language, and culture. It affirms that we are all part of a larger tapestry, interconnected in our shared humanity and responsibility to build a better future for those coming after us.

To conclude, I am grateful for you, my reader. I am grateful that you have trusted me with your time, the time you invested in my thoughts via these pages. I'm grateful that you care and hopeful you'll remember the words I began this book with:

"Speak up for those who cannot speak for themselves, for the rights of all who are destitute. Speak up and judge fairly; defend the rights of the poor and needy." -Proverbs 31: 8-9

My prayer for you is continued meaning and purpose in your work. I pray you find joy and satisfaction as you contribute to the betterment of civilization in healthcare and beyond. I pray the good Lord brings us to a place of love, peace, and generosity towards one another, understanding that we may not always agree with each other's viewpoints. I pray the Lord's will, be completed in all our lives.

With Love,

Dr. Dale

Interested in having Dr. Dale discuss this book with your audience?

Visit www.DoctorDaleMD.com to request him as a speaker.

More Books By Dr. Dale...

How to Raise a Doctor

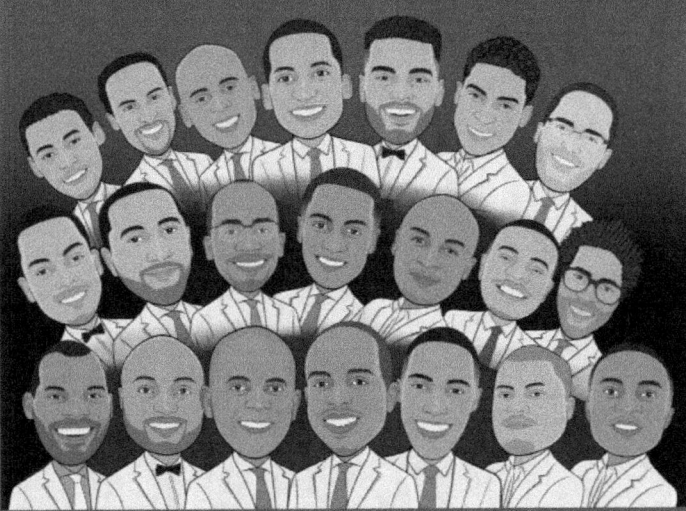

Black Men In White Coats

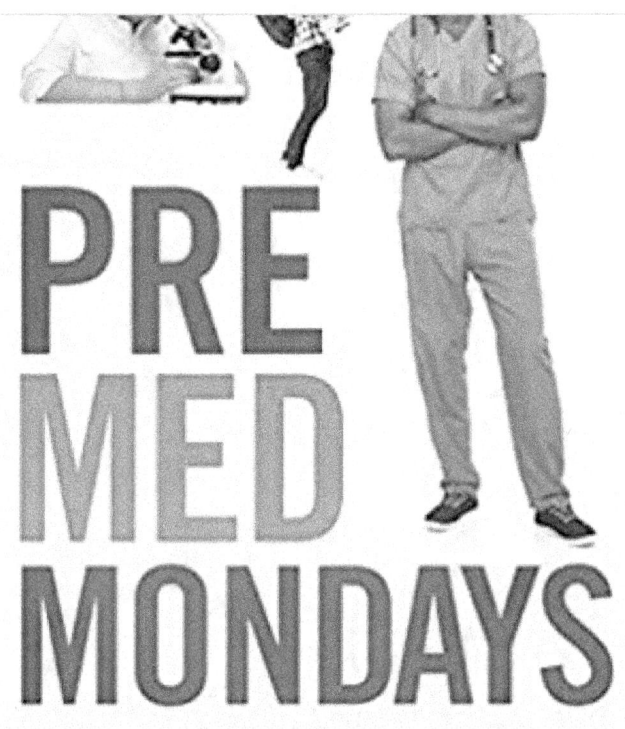

PRE MED MONDAYS

52 Letters of Mentorship to a Future Doctor

DALE OKORODUDU, MD

PreMed Mondays

A DOCTOR'S GUIDE TO

SELF-PUBLISHING

How to Become an Author and Influencer in Your Field

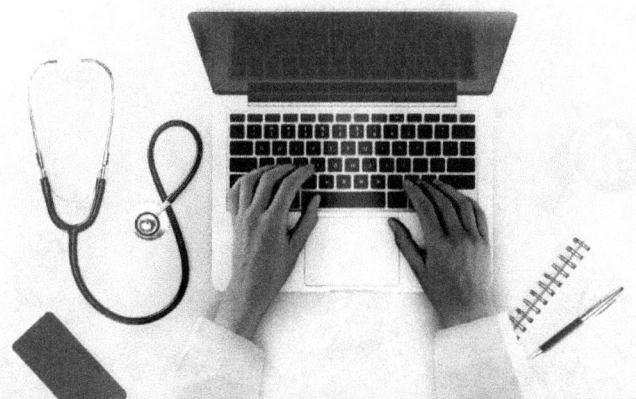

DALE OKORODUDU, MD

A Doctor's Guide to Self-Publishing

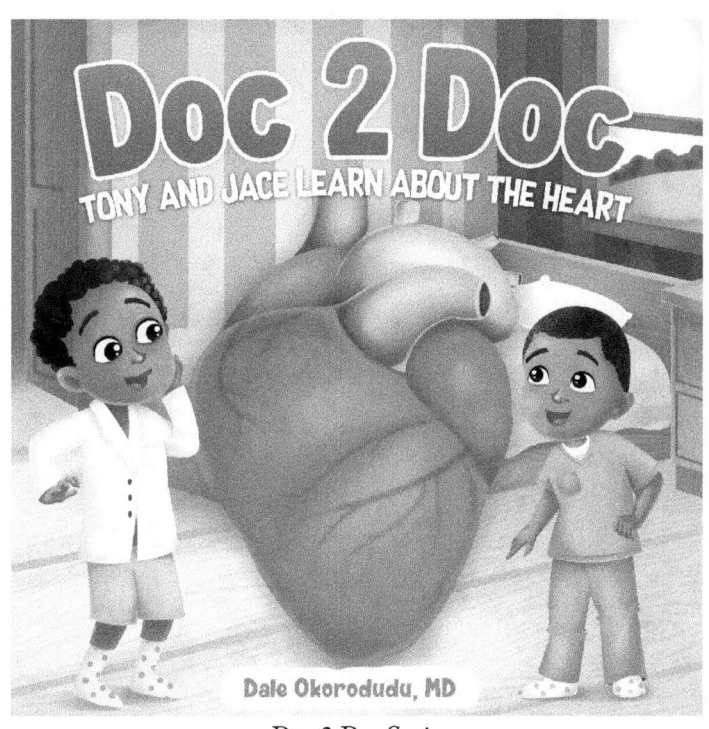

Doc 2 Doc Series

www.DoctorDaleMD.com